GASTRIC BYPASS SURGERY

PROCEDURES, BENEFITS AND HEALTH RISKS

SURGERY - PROCEDURES, COMPLICATIONS, AND RESULTS

Additional books in this series can be found on Nova's website
under the Series tab.

Additional e-books in this series can be found on Nova's website
under the e-book tab.

SURGERY - PROCEDURES, COMPLICATIONS, AND RESULTS

GASTRIC BYPASS SURGERY

PROCEDURES, BENEFITS AND HEALTH RISKS

EUGENE MONTGOMERY
EDITOR

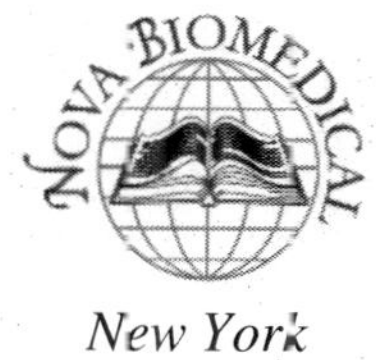

Nova Biomedical

New York

Copyright © 2016 by Nova Science Publishers, Inc.

All rights reserved. No part of this book may be reproduced, stored in a retrieval system or transmitted in any form or by any means: electronic, electrostatic, magnetic, tape, mechanical photocopying, recording or otherwise without the written permission of the Publisher.

We have partnered with Copyright Clearance Center to make it easy for you to obtain permissions to reuse content from this publication. Simply navigate to this publication's page on Nova's website and locate the "Get Permission" button below the title description. This button is linked directly to the title's permission page on copyright.com. Alternatively, you can visit copyright.com and search by title, ISBN, or ISSN.

For further questions about using the service on copyright.com, please contact:
Copyright Clearance Center
Phone: +1-(978) 750-8400   Fax: +1-(978) 750-4470   E-mail: info@copyright.com.

NOTICE TO THE READER

The Publisher has taken reasonable care in the preparation of this book, but makes no expressed or implied warranty of any kind and assumes no responsibility for any errors or omissions. No liability is assumed for incidental or consequential damages in connection with or arising out of information contained in this book. The Publisher shall not be liable for any special, consequential, or exemplary damages resulting, in whole or in part, from the readers' use of, or reliance upon, this material. Any parts of this book based on government reports are so indicated and copyright is claimed for those parts to the extent applicable to compilations of such works.

Independent verification should be sought for any data, advice or recommendations contained in this book. In addition, no responsibility is assumed by the publisher for any injury and/or damage to persons or property arising from any methods, products, instructions, ideas or otherwise contained in this publication.

This publication is designed to provide accurate and authoritative information with regard to the subject matter covered herein. It is sold with the clear understanding that the Publisher is not engaged in rendering legal or any other professional services. If legal or any other expert assistance is required, the services of a competent person should be sought. FROM A DECLARATION OF PARTICIPANTS JOINTLY ADOPTED BY A COMMITTEE OF THE AMERICAN BAR ASSOCIATION AND A COMMITTEE OF PUBLISHERS.

Additional color graphics may be available in the e-book version of this book.

Library of Congress Cataloging-in-Publication Data

ISBN: 978-1-63485-412-2
Library of Congress Control Number: 2016940995

Published by Nova Science Publishers, Inc. † New York

CONTENTS

PREFACE

Obesity is a multifactorial global epidemic with associated risk factors for an array of vascular, metabolic, psychological and economical consequences. Bariatric surgery has revealed a significant link between gastrointestinal metabolism and obesity that extends to resolution of many metabolic diseases including type 2 diabetes and cardiovascular disease risk. Bariatric surgery offers the most effective results and Roux-en Y gastric bypass (RYGB) is the most commonly performed bariatric surgery worldwide. The effective weight loss achieved by RYGB is thought to be caused by the re-arrangement of the gastrointestinal tract leading malabsorption and restriction of the ingested nutrients, and consequently resulting in alterations in the gut hormone levels. The first chapter of this book briefly summarizes the current literature on the changes in the gastrointestinal hormones following RYGB. Chapter Two studies the role of bariatric surgery in the resolution of obesity and type 2 diabetes. Chapter Three discusses how to treat a type 2 diabetic patient post-bariatric surgery. The last chapter discusses the recent findings of the relationship between gastric bypass and four different skin disorders.

In: Gastric Bypass Surgery
Editor: Eugene Montgomery

ISBN: 978-1-63485-412-2
© 2016 Nova Science Publishers, Inc.

Chapter 1

GASTROINTESTINAL HORMONES AND ROUX-EN-Y GASTRIC BYPASS

Deniz Atalayer, PhD
Sabancı University, Istanbul, Turkey

ABSTRACT

Obesity is a multifactorial global epidemic with associated risk factors for an array of vascular, metabolic, psychological and economical consequences. Bariatric surgery offers the most effective results and Roux-en-Y gastric bypass (RYGB) is the most commonly performed bariatric surgery worldwide. The effective weight loss achieved by RYGB is thought to be caused by the re-arrangement of the gastrointestinal tract leading malabsorption and restriction of the ingested nutrients, and consequently resulting in alterations in the gut hormone levels. This review briefly summarizes the current literature on the changes in the gastrointestinal hormones following RYGB. Understanding these post-operative alterations may provide insights on the efficacy of RYGB that may help developing superior surgical techniques, novel pharmacological and psychological interventions, as well as prevention strategies against obesity.

INTRODUCTION

Obesity is a global pandemic however; weight loss achieved by pharmacological and behavioral treatments are generally ineffective in maintaining a healthy body weight over a longer period of time and thus usually followed by weight regain. Bariatric surgery is currently the most effective anti-obesity intervention (Sjostrom et al., 2004, 2007) in comparison with the non-surgical treatments (Gloyet al., 2013; Buchwald et al., 2004) inducing a negative energy balance by reducing food intake (Rubino et al., 2010) and increasing energy expenditure (Stylopoulos et al., 2009). It also has been shown to improve glucose homeostasis and resolve type-2-diabetes (T2D) (Sala et al., 2014). Roux-en-Y gastric bypass (RYGB) has been the most commonly performed procedure in the world and although there had been a marked decrease in the number of RYGB performed from 2003 to 2008 with the co-morbid increase in the preference for sleeve gastrectomy, another bariatric surgery procedure, RYGB still remains the most commonly performed bariatric procedure worldwide in 2013 (Buchwald et al., 2009b, Angrisani et al., 2015).

During RYGB, a small proximal pouch (typically < 30 ml) is created from the stomach, which is attached to a segment of the jejunum that has been brought rostrally after being transected. The large gastric remnant is joined to the mid- to distal jejunum, creating the Roux-en-Y limb. RYGB causes restriction by reducing stomach capacity by ~95%, and re-directs the flow of nutrients, which results in ingested foods bypassing the 95% of the stomach, entire duodenum, and a small portion (15–20 cm) of the proximal jejunum (Cummings et al., 2004), passing the small re-sectioned stomach pouch directly being shunted into the mid- to distal jejunum. It has been reported that patients, after RYGB, often experience significant reductions in appetite, as well as greater satiety following the ingestion of smaller meals (Ashrafian et al., 2009). Several studies in humans and animals have shown that physiological changes in, i.e., intragastric pressure (Raybould 1991) and emptying rate (rats) (Kalogeris et al., 1983), as well as pyloric motility (Treacy et al., 1992), following nutrient delivery to different parts of the gastrointestinal (GI) tract. Moreover, the mechanoreceptors and chemoreceptors embedded in the lining of the GI tract respond to specific amount and type of macronutrients (Mei 1985). In RYGB, a re-arrangement of the GI tract is achieved; the nutrients bypass the duodenum and proximal jejunum and are being shunted directly into the mid jejunum. It is assumed that this re-arrangement causes alterations in the gut hormone responses, which may be contributing to the efficacy of RYGB on effecive weight loss (Cummings et al., 2004). However, the specific mechanisms underlying the efficacy of RYGB are still under investigation. It has been reported that RYGB produces changes in the gut-brain communication regulating energy balance which then leads to reductions in subjective appetite and food intake causing weight loss of approximately 25–30% of total body weight (Sjostrom et al., 2007). The weight loss following RYGB has been shown to plateau after 1-1.5 years and to be maintained in most patients for at least 10 years following the surgery (Sjostrom et al., 2007). However, the degree of successful weight loss after RYGB varies considerably along with the remission rates. Thus, understanding the hormonal changes following RYGB y may help elucidating the mechanisms underlying its success and lead to the development of novel preventative strategies and treatments with or without the surgical interventions.

GASTRIC SIGNALS

Gastrin, ghrelin and obestatin that are secreted by the stomach will be reviewed in this section.

Gastrin

Gastrin, a peptide of 34 amino acids, is secreted by G-cells that are located in the pyloric antrum and duodenum. It leads to the production of pepsinogen (an enzyme that breaks down the proteins) and stimulation of acid secretion in response to the expansion of the stomach or ingestion of protein, caffeine, and alcohol (Posovszky and Wabitsch 2015). A direct anorectic or orexigenic effect of gastrin is not established so far. Earlier studies showed significantly reduced gastrin release postprandially at 3 and 12 months following RYGB (Schrumpf et al., 1981). Recent data also indicated lower postprandial incremental area under the curve (iAUC) with no changes for fasting levels of gastrin at 2 weeks post-RYGB (Jacobsen et al., 2012). Postprandial reductions in gastrin levels were also reported following a protein-rich meal in RYGB patients after ≥ 3 months post-operativelyGrong et al., 2015). Moreover significant reductions in gastrin cells in the excluded portion of the stomach in RYGB patients compared to the obese controls (Safatle-Ribeiro et al., 2013) have been reported at ≥ 3 years of follow-up. Taken together, these reports, along with similar findings from animal studies (Stenstrom et al., 2006), suggest a reduction in gastrin levels following RYGB.

Ghrelin

Ghrelin has been shown to be a major orexigenic hormone, mainly produced by the endocrine X/A-cells of the oxyntic glands of the stomach mucosa and released to the blood stream (Choi et al., 2003; Sakata et al., 2009; Thompson et al., 2004). Studies have also shown that its expression is highest in the stomach (Kojima et al., 1999) and to a lesser degree, in the pituitary gland (Howard et al., 1996) and the hypothalamus (Wren et al., 2000). Ghrelin rises prior to meals and declines rapidly postprandially (Carlson et al., 2009; English et al., 2002; Zwirska-Korczala et al., 2007), suggesting a role in preprandial hunger and meal initiation (Cummings et al., 2001). Moreover, ghrelin has been shown to have a circadian fluctuation in both animals and humans; it increases in the morning and decreases later in the day. Conditions of positive energy balance (e.g., hyperglycemia, insulin resistance, obesity) are associated with lower ghrelin concentrations (Shiiya et al., 2002; Tschop et al., 2001). Obese individuals have lower fasting plasma ghrelin levels compared to lean people (Shiiya et al., 2002; Tschop et al., 2001). However, the reduced levels of ghrelin in obese individuals do not appear to prevent further weight gain. The lower fasting ghrelin levels in obesity suggest a possible down-regulation of ghrelin in response to overeating or excess body weight. Higher ghrelin levels, on the other hand, have been observed during periods of fasting, hunger, or other conditions associated with negative energy balance, such as short-term starvation, cancer cachexia, as well as anorexia nervosa (Bloomgarden, 2007).

The major hypothesis regarding the success behind the RYGB had been the suppression of the secretion of the main orexigenic hormone ghrelin (ghrelin hypothesis) (Cummings et al., 2002). This was supported by the majority of the studies showing decreases in ghrelin levels following the surgery (Foschi et al., 2008; Frühbeck et al., 2004; Garcia de la Torre et al., 2008; Lin et al., 2004; Morinigo et al., 2004; Rodieux et al., 2008). However, results have been inconsistent; increases (Pardina et al., 2009; Holdstock et al., 2003; Vendrell et al., 2004, Garcia-Fuentes et al. 2008) as well as no change (Korner et al., 2009; Whitson et al., 2007a) in ghrelin levels have also been reported.

It is important to note that there are two major molecular forms of ghrelin; octanoylated (acyl) which comprises <10% of circulating ghrelin, and des-n-octanoyl (des-acyl) ghrelin, which have different, and perhaps opposing functions in relation to energy homeostasis (Toshinai et al., 2006; Zhang et al., 2005). Although the des-acyl form of ghrelin comprises more than 90% of the total ghrelin released (Hosoda et al., 2000; Leite-Moreira and Soares, 2007), the acyl (active ghrelin) is the portion that binds to the growth hormone secretagogue receptor-1A (Kojima et al., 1999) to regulate several metabolic processes and to promote food intake. Thus, it had become crucial to analyze the total, acyl and des-acyl ghrelin separately and therefore the assays distinguishing between acyl and des-acyl ghrelin moieties have been developed recently (Prudom et al., 2010). The reports using such assays support the initial ghrelin hypothesis showing significant reductions in the fasting levels of total and active ghrelin as well as postprandial (AUC) levels of active ghrelin at 2 weeks following RYGB (Jacobsen et al., 2012). Fasting and postprandial (AUC) des-acyl ghrelin levels were also shown to decrease in RYGB patients at 1-year follow-up (Nannipieri et al., 2013). Interestingly, studies indicated that both fasting and postprandial (AUC) total ghrelin levels following 1 and 3 months returned to pre-surgery levels at 1-year post-surgery follow-up (Peterliet al., 2012). Increases at 1-year post-op following an initial decrease have been consistently reported for total, active and des-acyl ghrelin during fasting and postprandially (Sundbom et al., 2007; Samat et al., 2013; Yang et al., 2014). It is possible that ghrelin decreases are transient after RYGB; and that ghrelin subsequently increases as weight loss continues due to lower food intake.

Obestatin

Obestatin is a 23-amino acid peptide hormone and is derived from posttranslational cleavage of preproghrelin, and released from the stomach (Zhang et al., 2005; Zhao et al., 2008). Although ghrelin is an orexigenic hormone, obestatin has been shown to have anorexigenic effects such as reducing food intake, delaying gastric emptying, and reducing body weight in rodents therefore antagonizing the orexigenic effect of ghrelin (Zhang et al., 2005). However, later, controversial findings have been reported on the effects of obestatin on food intake (Gourcerol et al., 2007; Lacquaniti et al., 2011). In humans, the common finding was that the fasting plasma obestatin was to be reduced in obese individuals compared to the normal-weight persons (Lippl et al., 2008; Huda et al., 2008; Guo et al., 2007) along with the findings showing lower ghrelin-to-obestatin ratio in obese vs. normal weight women (Vicennati et al., 2007). A study reported a significant decrease in obestatin levels after a gastrectomy surgery (Huda et al., 2008) and studies investigating the changes in obestatin levels following RYGB have mostly been contraversial reporting increases at 1-year (Yang et al., 2014) and 3-year (Martins et al., 2011), as well as no change at 2-year follow-ups (Roth et al., 2009).

FOREGUT SIGNALS

In this section, cholecystokinin (CCK) and glucose-dependent insulinotropic peptide (GIP) that are secreted by the duodenum and jejunum will be reviewed.

Cholecystokinin (CCK)

CCK was the first gut hormone found to be implicated in appetite control (Gibbs et al., 1973). It regulates gut motility, pancreatic secretion, and gall bladder contractions. It is secreted predominately from the I-cells in the duodenum and jejunum in response to the presence of nutrients in the intestinal lumen (Lieverse et al., 1994, Parker et al., 2005, Liddle et al., 1985). CCK regulates the digestive enzymes from the pancreas, stimulates gall bladder contraction, increases intestinal motility and inhibits gastric emptying (Liddle et al., 1985, Moran et al., 1994). Higher concentrations are associated with a reduction in meal size and meal duration. CCK has a short plasma half-life of a few minutes, plasma levels of CCK rise within 15 minutes after meal ingestion (Liddle et al., 1985) and enhance perceptions of fullness and reduce hunger during the course of a meal in both humans and animals (Kissilef et al., 1981; 2003; Gibbs et al., 1973). Fatty acids (with chain lengths of 12 or more carbons) and proteins stimulate CCK secretion (Holzer et al., 1994; Lal et al., 2004; Corp et al., 2003). It has been suggested that CCK signaling is a vagally mediated process between the gut and the brain. Supporting this, studies with animals showed that vagotomised rats do not show the lipid induced delay in gastric emptying or suppression in subsequent food intake (Moriarty et al., 1997). Moreover it has been shown that there is CCK-1 receptor expression in human vagal afferent neurons (Feinle et al., 2003).

Although CCK is involved in meal-termination, it does not appear to have an independent role in the long-term regulation of energy balance and body weight, but rather a primary role in short term control of appetite and satiety (Moran, 2000; Tadross and le Roux 2009). Thus, there had not been much interest in investigating CCK regarding a possible role in the efficacy of RYGB and are only few studies to date reporting on the changes in CCK levels following RYGB. Earlier studies compared postprandial CCK levels following RYBG showed that the CCK response was not affected (Rubino et al., 2004; Kellum et al., 1990). In addition, animal studies also lead similar findings: CCK was not significantly altered after RYGB-induced weight loss in rats, (Suzuki et al., 2005). However recent studies suggested some effects, at 1-week (Peterli et al., 2012) and 2-weeks (Jacobsen et al., 2012) following the surgery: the patients with RYGB had elevated postprandial maximum peak CCK levels with no difference for AUC concentrations. Thus, postprandial CCK peak was increased, but the effect was short-lasting. Post-operative fasting CCK levels were also shown to be unchanged (Jacobsen et al., 2012). Although a reduction in CCK following RYGB might be expected due to the diversion of the ingested food away from it secretion site -the upper part of the small intestine (the duodenum), the jejunum also was shown to release CCK (Katsusuke et al., 2008), whichmay explain the unchanged AUC levels of CCK following surgery. However, the role of CCK in the efficiency of RYGB warrants further investigations.

Glucose-Dependent Insulinotropic Peptide (GIP)

Glucose-dependent insulinotropic polypeptide (GIP) is a 42 amino acid peptide and is proposed to have a role in the pathophysiology of obesity and type-2-diabetes (T2D). It is one of two well-known incretins (along with glucagon-like peptide-1; GLP-1) and synthesized in the enteroendocrine cells (K-cells) primarily in the proximal small intestine (duodenum and jejunum) and its secretion is induced by food intake, especially carbohydrate and lipid intake (Nauck, 1986). Once released, GIP stimulates β-cells of the Islets of Langerhans to cause GIP secretion which gives it the property of an incretin. It also inhibits gastric acid secretion, suppresses lipolysis in adipose tissue, induces appetite and reduces energy expenditure in the brain (Paschetta et al., 2011). It promotes glucose absorption in the small intestine by increasing the number of GLUT1 glucose receptors (Creutzfeldt et al., 2001; Cheeseman 1996, 1998) and based on its effects on insulin secretion, GIP has been offered as a critical target for T2D treatments and etiology. Several studies have found that GIP (both basal and simulated) was elevated in obese compared to lean persons (Vilsboll et al., 2003) and severely blunted in patients with T2D (Saxena et al., 2010; Gautier et al., 2008).

In an RYGB procedure, the duodenum and a part of the jejunum are bypassed resulting in a lack of nutrient exposure (Rao and Kini, 2011). This rationale was agreed with the proponents of the foregut theory explaining the efficacy of RYGB, whereby bypass of the proximal small intestine leads to decreased anti-incretin effects. Thus, less GIP secretion was predicted following RYGB (Pories and Albrecht, 2001; Rubino 2008). However, results have been less consistent, with studies showing elevated (Lafarrere et al., 2007; 2008; Goldfine et al., 2007) or reduced (Rodieux et al., 2008; Korner et al., 2007), as well as unchanged GIP levels independent of weight loss (Cohen et al., 2007). Fasting GIP levels were reduced in diabetics but no change in non-diabetics who underwent RYGB at a 3-week (Rubino et al., 2004) as well as at 6- and 12-week (Clements et al., 2004) follow-ups. Furthermore, no change in non-fasting plasma GIP levels at 6-month follow-up in diabetic and non-diabetic RYGB patients have also been reported (Whitson et al., 2007a). Similarly, total postprandial iAUC GIP levels over a 4-hour period were significantly reduced in the non-diabetic RYGB patients compared to the gastric banding and non-operated controls (Rodieux et al., 2008) $\geq$ 9-48 months after the surgery The most recent study by Xiong et al. (2015) showed that fasting and postprandial (at the 2-hour point) GIP decreased following RYGB at the 1-week and 1, 3, and 6-month follow-up periods gradually. However one limitation of this study is that in their sample they used a group of gastric cancer patients with T2D and or simple T2D. Thus their report may not be representative of non-diabetic obese nor T2D patients. However, in diabetic RYGB patients at a 1-month follow-up, postprandial GIP was found to increase 1.5 fold in response to 50g glucose load (Laferrere et al., 2007; 2008). Another study also reported plasma GIP increases in hypoglycemic vs. non-hypoglycemic RYGB patients in response to a standard test meal (Rabiee et al., 2011). A possible explanation for the inconsistencies in the literature may stem from the nature of the GIP action. During this peak, the major insulinotropic effect of GIP is achieved at approximately 60 min after an oral glucose bolus and serum levels return to basal levels in approximately 120–180 min (Nauck, 1986). The short half life of GIP (Nauck, 1986) as well as the fast degradation following its peak after a bolus with only a small percentage left in the circulation however makes the detection and analyses of GIP in serum extremely difficult as well as unreliable. One group used whole blood

GIP mRNA as a marker for systemic GIP gene expression to avoid the unreliability issues of measuring serum GIP (Moran-Atkin et al., 2013). In agreement with Lafarere et al.'s (2007; 2008) findings, they showed significant increases in GIP gene expression in correlation with the clinical amelioration of T2D following RYGB (Moran-Atkin et al., 2013). To summarize, the current literature suggests that GIP levels are elevated in persons with obesity and T2D which may contribute to insulin resistance and defective glucose-stimulated insulin secretion that are symptomatic in these conditions. Along with this, majority of the findings seems to agree with the notion that GIP decreases following RYGB. Thus, GIP antagonism may be considered a target action for the therapeutic agents as decrease in GIP or a blockade in its action seem to be theoretically and preliminarily useful for obese persons and T2D patients. However, inconsistencies warrant further investigation.

HIND GUT SIGNALS

L cell-derived factors (peptide tyrosine tyrosine (PYY), glucagon like peptide-1 (GLP-1), GLP- 2, oxyntomodulin (OXM)), pancreatic signals (pancreatic polypeptide (PP), glucagon, insulin, amylin, somatostatin), and adipokines (leptin, adiponectin, resistin) will be reviewed in this section. GLP-1, GLP-2, OXM along with the pancreatic glucagon are products of proglucagon gene and known as proglucagon-derived peptides. However post-translational processing of proglucagon-derived peptides differs in a tissue-specific manner: glucagon is the main product in the pancreas, whereas GLP-1, GLP-2, OXM are the major products in the intestine and the brain (Posovszky and Wabitsch, 2015a; 2015b). PYY (PYY_{1-36} and PYY_{3-36}) and PP almost exclusively expressed at the level of the digestive system (Cox, 2007; Holzer et al., 2012).

L Cell-Derived Factors

Intestinal L cells are open-type cells predominantly located in the distal ileum and colon and express fatty acid receptors (Pozowski and Wabitsch, 2015a). GLP-1, GLP-2, and OXM are cleaved from the precursor preproglucagon that is synthesized from the intestinal L cells along with PYY. Together, the L cell-derived factors are thought to meadiate an ileal brake effect by reducing gastric acid secretion, gastric emptying and decelerating mouth-to-cecum transit time, and thus reduce food intake and prevent malabsorption and postprandial metabolic disturbances.

Peptide Tyrosine Tyrosine (PYY$_{3-36}$)

PYY is a 36-amino-acid peptide that has two circulating endogenous forms (PYY$_{1-36}$ and PYY$_{3-36}$) and is one of the Neuropeptide Y peptide family, along with Y (NPY), and pancreatic polypeptide (PP) (Michel, 1998; Cox, 2007). PYY$_{3-36}$ is the biologically active form (Batterham et al., 2003a) and originally isolated from porcoine intestine (Tatemoto, 1982). It is produced mostly in the small intestine and colon, released from the L-cells of the distal small bowel postprandially in proportion to the consumed calories. It is co-localized with pro-glucagon products, glicentin and glucagon-like peptide 1 (GLP-1) and GLP-2 (Ekblad and Sunder, 2002). It inhibits food intake (Batterham et al., 2002), increases energy expenditure (Guo et al., 2006) and delays gastric emptying (Sloth et al., 2007). PYY immunoreactivity is also found in the central nervous system regions such as the hypothalamus, medulla, pons, and spinal cord (Ekblad and Sundler, 2002; Kara et al., 2009). G-protein coupled Y receptor superfamily (Y1, Y2, Y4, Y5 and Y6) has specific affinities for each member of the peptide family; NPY and PYY do not grossly differ in their affinities for the Y1, Y2 and Y5 receptors subtypes and PYY$_{3-36}$ prefrentially binds to Y2 receptors (Cox, 2007). Endogenous PYY$_{3-36}$ levels were found to be low (Batterham et al., 2003a; Cummings et al., 2004; le Roux et al., 2006; Peterli et al., 2012) and blunted in obese individuals (Ashby and Bloom 2007), and increased in patients with anorexia nervosa (Misra et al., 2006).

Postprandial (AUC) PYY$_{3-36}$ levels were persistently elevated post-operatively at 2 weeks (Evans et al., 2012), at 1-month (Jacobsen et al., 2012), and 3- and 12-month follow-ups (Korner et al., 2009; Bose et al., 2010). At a 12-month follow-up, it has been reported that fasting and 3-meal (9-hour) postprandial PYY$_{3-36}$ (AUC) levels did not differ between patients who lost 85% of their initial weight compared to the patients who only lost 35% of their initial weight (Dirksen et al., 2013a). However both group of patients had higher levels of AUC PYY$_{3-36}$ than the normal weight individuals showing that the increased levels of PYY$_{3-36}$ did not correlate with weight loss following surgery (Dirksen et al., 2013a). Similarly, postprandial peak for PYY$_{3-36}$ and AUC analysis for postprandialPYY$_{3-36}$ were found to increase significantly in

RYGB patients at 1-month follow-up at 10% weight loss compared to the dieting group with the equivalent weight loss (approx. at 8 weeks) (Lafarrere et al., 2010). Regarding the fasting levels of PYY_{3-36} several studies reported no change following RYGB at 2-week (Evans et al., 2012) and 1-year (Bose et al., 2010) follow-ups, and with 7-10% weight loss (Plum et al., 2011). These implicate that the effect of RYGB on PYY_{3-36} is not weight loss dependent and is possibly related to the re-arrangement of the GI tract.

Glucagon Like Peptide-1 (GLP-1)

GLP-1 is mainly released by the L-cells of the small bowel following meal ingestion (Naslund et al., 2004; Feinle et al., 2003; Hermann et al., 1995; Doyle and Egan, 2007; Jang et al., 2007).) There are multiple circulating moieties of GLP-1: the biologically active forms, $GLP-1_{7-37}$ (comprising the 80% of the circulating GLP-1) and $GLP-1_{7-36}$ and the inactive forms $GLP-1_{1-37}$ and $GLP-1_{1-36}$. The active forms are powerful insulinotropics (i.e., they induce insulin secretion) (Schmidt et al., 1985). They act on the pancreas to secrete insulin (incretin effect) and also slow gastric emptying, inhibit glucagon release (Komatsu et al., 1989; Willms et al., 1996, Russell-Jones and Gough, 2012). GLP-1 is secreted in two phases; the first short rapid release occurs 5-10 minutes following a meal, and the later delayed and extended release occurs 30 to 60 minutes postprandially (Hermann et al., 1995; Ghatei et al., 1983). Thus, it is hypothesized that there are two distinct mechanisms of GLP-1 secretion. The initial phase occurs when L-cells and K/L cells in the upper small intestine are in contact with the nutrients whereas the prolonged second phase occurs when L-cells in the distal bowel are activated (Rocca and Brubaker, 1999; De León et al., 2006). Thus, GLP-1 along with PYY may contribute to the "ileal brake" (Wen et al., 1995), an inhibitory feedback process of nutrients (specifically lipids) in the colon inhibiting motility and transit of further nutrients within the upper GI tract to optimize the meal digestion and absorption (Spiller et al., 1984).

Post-operatively, enhanced amounts of postprandial circulating GLP-1(both maximum peak and AUC) with no change in the fasting levels, have been repeatedly shown, even when there is no significant weight loss (Peterli et al., 2009; Karamanakos et al., 2012; Bose et al., 2010; Borg et al., 2006; Morinigo et al., 2006; 2008; le Roux et al., 2007; Korner et al., 2006; 2007; 2009; Laferrère et al., 2008; 2010; de Carvalho et al., 2009; Goldfine et al., 2007; Dirksen et al., 2010; Holdstock et al., 2008; Ochner et al., 2011).

Furthermore, increased GLP-1 receptor signaling and GLP-1 secretion from the L-cells have also been shown (Mason, 1999; Gaitonde et al., 2012). The reduced size of the stomach and exclusion of the foregut, together allow for a faster delivery of food contents through the gut which may add to the dramatic increase in GLP-1 levels following RYGB. This is the 'hindgut' mechanism that has been proposed in explaining the efficacy of RYGB, whereby a direct flow nutrients to the distal small bowel causing an increase in the incretin effect. Thus the elevated levels of GLP-1 may contribute to the successful weight loss following RYGB in addition to the glucose homeostasis-related effects (i.e.T2D improvements and resolution) (Laferrère et al., 2008; Bose et al., 2009; Peterli et al., 2009). Based on these reports, it is likely that an earlier and enhanced increase in postprandial GLP-1 (and PYY_{3-36}) levels after RYGB may contribute to an early sense of satiety and reduced meal size (Santoro et al., 2008; Borg et al., 2006; le Roux et al., 2006; Rodieux et al., 2008) regardless of the reported unchanged fasting levels in both hormones.

Glucagon-Like Peptide-2 (GLP-2)

The 33-amino-acid peptide GLP-2, along with GLP-1, is also cleaved from the precursor proglucagon by intestinal endocrine L-cells (Rothenberg et al., 1995). However, unlike GLP-1, GLP-2 is not insulinotropic; does not inhibit insulin, but it is co-secreted with GLP-1 into the bloodstream in response to ingestion of lipids and proteins (Doyle and Egan, 2007; Jang et al., 2007; Matikainen et al., 2016). GLP-2 reduces gastric motility and acid secretion (Burrin et al., 2001), increases hexose transport, and in animals is shown to inhibit feeding (Tang-Christensen et al., 2000; Rotondo et al., 2011). However, there are only few studies to date that examined the changes in GLP-2 following bariatric surgery. In a study with obese persons with T2D, GLP-2 was shown to significantly increase postprandially (AUC) 6-weeks after RYGB (Romero et al., 2012). Another study comparing RYGB patients who are weight loss resistant and surgery patients achieving successful weight loss showed no changes in the fasting and postprandial (AUC) levels of GLP-2 at 1-year follow-up (de Hollanda et al., 2014). However, although a statistical significance was not reached, an increasing trend for postprandial (AUC) GLP-2 was noted for the successful weight loss group (1354 ± 256 ng/mL) vs. weight loss resistant patients (658 ± 341 ng/mL, marginal means ± SD) (de Hollanda et al., 2014). Increased plasma GLP-2 was also shown following RYGB operation in rats (Le Roux et al., 2010). Based on its role in initiating intestinal epithelial barrier function and mucosal growth (Burrin et al., 2001; Holst 2010) GLP-2 may play a role in gut adaptation following RYGB to prevent malabsorption (Rhee et al., 2015).

Oxyntomodulin (OXM)

OXM is a 37-amino acid peptide originally isolated from porcine jejunoileal cells (Bataille et al., 1981). It is released from the gut in post-prandial state thus has anorectic effects. OXM is another product of the preproglucagon gene and is co-secreted with GLP-1 and PYY by the L-cells of the distal intestines, in response to nutrient ingestion proportionally to the calorie intake (Ghatei et al., 1983). Laferrere and colleagues (2010) also showed that the increase of OXM was strongly correlated with total GLP-1 and PYY_{3-36} after gastric bypass surgery. It was found that OXM shows glucagon-like activity in the liver (Bataille et al., 1982) and has a much lower potency when compared with GLP-1 (Schjoldager et al., 1988). OXM also inhibits gastric acid secretion and delays gastric emptying (Schjoldager et al., 1989). Administration of OXM is associated with decreased food intake and increased energy expenditure in both rodents and humans (Dakin et al., 2001; Cohen et al., 2003; Wynne et al.; 2006, Maida et al., 2008).

Recently, few groups have investigated OXM levels following RYGB. Laferrere and colleagues (2010) reported enhanced levels of OXM (AUC and maximum peak) in response to oral glucose tolerance test (OGTT; 50g glucose load) 1-month following RYGB in morbidly obese women with T2D, which was not found in patients who achieved an equivalent weight loss by dieting. (Laferrere et al., 2010). A similar result was also reported by Le Roux and colleagues showing OXM increases following a standard breakfast postprandially (AUC) 6 months after RYGB (Werling et al., 2015). Another group have also reported slight OXM increases at 2- and 4-months following RYGB for postprandial levels (AUC) in response to OGTT and during fasting, however the effects were not statistically significant (Wu et al., 2013).

The proglucagon gene is also expressed in the intestines L-cells where it is cleaved into a number of peptides other than glucagon (i.e., GLP-1, GLP-2, OXM, glicentin) which were originally termed "enteroglucagon," and are collectively known as "proglucagon-derived peptides." Previous studies indicate that OXM makes up 30–40% of the plasma concentration of enteroglucagon in humans (Holst et al., 1983). Glicentin is a product of the proglucagon gene, and part of it is cleaved to generate OXM similar to GLP-1

(Sinclair and Drucker, 2005; Sala et al., 2014) and some researchers consider glicentin only a remnant metabolite of proglucagon after the cleavage of GLP-1 and GLP-2 (Sinclair and Drucker, 2005). Falken et al. (2011) reported a progressive rise in enteroglucagon at 3 days, 2 months, and 1 year following RYGB. Thus Falken et al. (2011) suggested that OXM may play an indirect role in the consequent weight loss.

PANCREATIC SIGNALS

The pancreatic endocrine cells are located in islets of Langerhans that contain four principal cell types, and are defined by the hormones they secrete. These include insulin and amylin-secreting β-cells (70%), glucagon-secreting α-cells (20%), somatostatin-secreting δ-cells, and pancreatic polypeptide–secreting PP-cells (originally termed F cells) (Fiocca et al., 1983).

Glucagon

Glucagon is produced by α-cells in the pancreatic islets of Langerhans and once released, binds to glucagon receptors in the liver initiating its critical role in glucose homeostasis by increasing glycogenolysis and gluconeogenesis (Dunning et al., 2007). Glucagon, along with the intestinal GLP-1, GLP-2, OXM, glicentin, is synthesized initially as the protein proglucagon, which, in mammals, is encoded by a single gene. Decreases in food intake have been shown following glucagon administration both in animals (Martin and Novin, 1977) and humans (Penick and Hinkle 1961; Grossman 1986; Geary et al., 1992). It has been used as a therapeutic agent to treat severe hypoglycemia due to excess exogenous insulin administration, neonatal hyperinsulinism (Aynsley-Green et al., 2000), tumor-induced hypoglycemia (Chung et al., 1996), and severe post-RYGB hypoglycemia (Halperin et al., 2010). Elevated fasting plasma glucagon concentrations have been reported in severely obese individuals (Swarbrick et al., 2008).

Although the role of glucagon in glucose homeostasis is well established, so far the relationship between gut hormone responses and glucagon level changes following RYGB has not been extensively studied. Following RYGB (1-4 weeks post-surgery), fasting glucagon was reported to slightly increase (Swarbrick et al., 2008; Jacobsen et al., 2012; Jorgensen et al., 2012). Postprandial (with mixed meal text) glucagon has been found to be significantly higher 2 weeks following RYGB compared to the preoperative levels (Jacobsen et al., 2012) whereas this difference has not been found for glucose tolerance tests (25g and 50g). Lafarere et al. (2010) however found significant increases for AUC analysis of postprandial (OGTT; 50g glucose) glucagon at 1-month follow-up in RYGB patients compared to the dieting group with the equivalent weight loss (8 weeks). Using a mixed meal test, Campos et al. (2013) also reported that postprandial (AUC) glucagon increased at 2 weeks post-operatively however this did not persist and returned to the preoperative baseline levels at 6 months following RYGB. Similar results came from Jorgensen et al. (2012) showing postprandial (mixed meal) increases at 1 week after RYGB which declined and returned to the baseline levels at 3- and 12-month follow-ups. Another study in obese patients with T2D also confirmed these findings that, fasting and postprandial (AUC) glucagon increased 2-4 weeks following RYGB which returned to baseline levels at 3-, 6-, and 12- month follow-ups (Swarbrick et al., 2008; Nannipieri et al., 2013). However, in an earlier study, glucagon values were still found to be higher during mixed meal test in RYGB patients after 2-4 years following the surgerycompared to the obese controls (Goldfine et al., 2007). It should be noted that Goldfine et al. (2007) used a cross-sectional study design study that may affect the results based on a possible lower baseline glucagon levels of the obese controls at the time of the study compared to the preoperative baseline glucagon levels in RYGB patients. Thus, based on the previous longitudinal studies, it is a stronger assumption that glucagon has an excursion at short-term after RYGB and a long-term decrease after a substantial weight loss.

Insulin

Insulin is one of the principal hormones involved in glucose metabolism and is synthesized in the ß-cells of the pancreas and rises rapidly after a meal, with well characterized optimization of glycaemic index (Polonsky et al., 1988). Insulin resistance −a key feature of T2D (along with the subsequent hypoinsulinemia followed by hyperglycemia) is defined as the reduced sensitivity to the metabolic actions of insulin on glucose homeostasis in the muscles and fat tissue or the suppressed hepatic glucose production in the liver (Rask-Madsen et al., 2012; Kahn et al., 2014). Insulin concentrations vary directly with body fat and insulin sensitivity is negatively correlated with body adiposity (Despres and Lemieux, 2006) and reductions of fasting insulin have been well documented following weight loss (Schwartz and Seeley, 1997).

RYGB has been suggested as a potential treatment for T2D as an alternative to pharmacological agents and meta-analyses and longitudinal studies report that that 60-80% of the RYGB patients show a complete resolution of T2D markers such as lower insulin sensitivity and resistance as well as blood glucose levels (Ferrannini et al., 2009; Buchwald et al., 2009a; Adams et al., 2012; Edholm et al., 2013; Yip et al., 2013). Fasting insulin and insulin resistance have been found to lower following RYGB in obese adults (Rodieux et al., 2008; Plum et al., 2011; Jacobsen et al., 2012; Peterli et al., 2009; 2012; Nannipieri et al., 2013) and adolescents (Oberbach et al., 2014). Postprandial (AUC) insulin following a mixed meal was shown to significantly decrease at 1-year follow-up whereas this was not shown at 2 weeks following the surgery (Nannipieri et al., 2013). However, Korner and colleagues reported greater insulin sensitivity and lower insulin resistance (HOMA-IR) following a intravenous glucose tolerance tests (IGTT) and fasting insulin levels in patients who underwent RYGB compared to persons who lost equal amount (7-10% weight loss) of weight by dieting (Plum et al., 2011). Campos et al. (2013) used a more accurate technique (Borai et al., 2011) of hyperinsulinemic euglycemic clamp to measure insulin sensitivity. They found that the average steady-state insulin concentration during the final hour of the euglycemic–hyperinsulinemic clamp decreased significantly in the morbidly obese non-diabetic RYGB patients 2-weeks after surgery, but was unchanged in the dieting group. Moreover, at the 6-month follow-up, when substantial weight loss has been reached, the decrease in steady-state insulin concentrations during clamp persisted, relative to pre-operative values (Campos et al., 2013). In agreement with this,1-year changes in insulin sensitivity were shown to correlate with the corresponding changes in body mass index (BMI) following RYGB (Nannipieri et al., 2013). Thus, the early changes seem to be weight loss-independent.

Pancreatic Polypeptide (PP)

PP, the other member of the Neuropeptide Y Fold Family, is synthesized by endocrine PP cells in the pancreatic islets of Langerhans. It is secreted in response to a meal (Ekblad and Sundler, 2002), exerting anorexic effects in humans (Batterham et al., 2003b) by a mechanism through the parasympathetic vagus nerve (Asakawa et al., 2003; Cox, 2007; Field et al.,

2010). The anorectic effects of PP are abolished by vagotomy in rodents (Asakawa et al., 2003). Its role in inhibits gastric emptying which may in part account for its ability to reduce appetite (Murphy and Bloom, 2006; Field et al., 2010).

In RYGB patients, fasting PP was shown to have a strong tendency to decrease at 2 weeks (Jacobsen et al., 2012; Campos et al., 2013), which was found to be significant at 1-month and 1-year follow-ups (Swarbrick et al., 2008). One study with T2D patients who underwent RYGB showed significant increases in fasting PP at 2-weeks which persisted at 1-year follow-up independent of the T2D remission (Nannipieri et al., 2013). However, the same study also showed marked reductions in postprandial (AUC) PP levels at both 2-week and 1-year follow-ups (Nannipieri et al., 2013). Others reported similar findings for non-T2D RYGB patients 2 weeks after the surgery (Swarbrick 2008; Campos et al., 2013) and at the 12-month follow-up (Dirksen et al., 2013a).

Amylin

Islet/insulinoma amyloid polypeptide (IAPP, amylin) is a 37-aminoacid secreted hormone that was discovered (Westermark et al., 1986) to be co-secreted with insulin from the in the β-cells within the pancreatic islets of Langerhans with a molar ratio of approximately 15:1 (insulin:amylin) (Hay et al., 2015) in response to blood glucose levels (Kahn et al., 1990). Amylin has been shown to inhibit insulin-stimulated glucose metabolism and muscle glycogen synthesis, and to slow gastric emptying (Hay et al., 2015). It is considered a satiety hormone (Lutz 2005) based on its short-term effects lowering food intake mainly via reducing meal sizes that is possibly through the central mechanisms within the hypothalamus and brain stem (Rowland et al., 1997; Lutz and Meyer 2015). Similar to leptin and insulin, number of experiments suggests a role for amylin as an adiposity signal affecting eating behavior by enhancing the anorectic effects of CCK (Mollet et al., 2003) and obesity was shown to be associated with high levels of amylin (Nannipieri et al., 2013). Administration of pramlintide, a synthetic analogue of human amylin, has been shown to improve glycaemic control and decrease body weight in T2D patients (Thompson et al., 1998; Schorr and Ofan, 2012; Weinzimer et al., 2012) suggesting a role for amylin in glucose mechanism and body weight regulation in humans.

Several studies reported decreased fasting and postprandial amylin (AUC) levels following RYGB at 1-year follow-up (Bose et al., 2010; Nannipieri et al., 2013). However reports on the 2-week follow-up have shown no change in amlyin levels (Nannipieri et al., 2013; Jacobsen et al., 2015). Bose et al., (2010) reported significantly reduced fasting and postprandial amlyin levels at the time when patients reached at least a weight loss of 12kg. These results seem to be in line with the notion that amylim may be considered an adiposity signal. Consistent with this, a recent study showed an association between BMI decreases and lower levels of total amylin in adolescents (Jensen et al., 2015). However most of the studies investigating amylin had been on preclinical models and further investigation is needed to fully understand its mechanism of action in humans.

Somatostatin

Somatostatin is mainly produced in the pancreas but also in the hypothalamus and in the D-cells of the GI tract exerting inhibitory functions and thus decreases the release of GI hormones and appetite (Barkan et al., 2003). Somatostatin analogs were shown to significantly reduce postprandial sensations of fullness in obese humans after a satiating meal without altering the tolerated maximum meal volume or postprandial gastric volume, suggesting an effect on the upper gut sensation but not directly on satiety regulation (Cremonini et al., 2005). Few studies assessing somatostatin showed no change following RYGB during a fasted state (Falken et al., 2011; Jacobsen et al., 2012) and postprandially (AUC) following an OGTT (50g glucose) or a mixed meal (Jacobsen et al., 2012). Statistical significance was reached for AUC levels in response to 25g glucose load for the same study (Jacobsen et al., 2012).

ADIPOKINES

The adipokines are cytokines that are secreted by the adipose tissue.Leptin was the first adipokine that was discovered (Zhang et al., 1994) and is released by the white adipose tissue (WAT).

Leptin

Leptin is an anorexigenic hormone and involved in long-term energy balance primarily by acting on the hypothalamus to decrease food intake and to increase energy expenditure (Beckman et al., 2011). It is secreted predominantly by the adipocytes with circulating levels proportionally to the fat mass in the body (Considine et al., 1996) and was observed to be higher in obese (vs. lean) persons during fasting and postprandially (Carlson et al., 2009; Carroll et al., 2007). Thus, perhaps it is not surprising that decreased leptin levels have consistently been reported following RYGB (Molina et al., 2003; Nijhuis et al., 2004; DePaula et al., 2009; Korner et al., 2009; Stoeckli et al., 2004; Kotidis et al., 2006; Shak et al., 2008; Faraj et al., 2003; Rubino et al., 2004; Lafarrere et al., 2010; Woelnerhanssen et al., 2011; Terra et al., 2013; Yousseif et al., 2014), and all bariatric surgeries irrespective of the surgery type (Frühbeck et al., 2002; Cigdem et al., 201; Knerr et al., 2006; Garcia de la Torre et al., 2008).

Adiponectin

Adiponectin or adipocyte complement–related protein of 30 kDa is a circulating protein and like leptin, secreted predominantly from the adipose tissue and is highly abundant in the plasma. However, unlike leptin, adiponectin levels remain relatively constant throughout the day and are not affected by food intake (Arora et al., 2006) and inversely correlated with body fat percentage in adults (Ukkola and Santaniemi, 2002) and BMI (Vendrell et al., 2004). Lower plasma levels of adiponectin have been reported in obese individuals with T2D compared to the non-diabetic obese individuals (Vendrell et al., 2004; Garcia de la Torre et al., 2008), suggesting a role in insulin resistance.

Following RYGB, adiponectin has been consistently shown to increase (Holdstock et al., 2003; Vendrell et al., 2004; Garcia de la Torre et al., 2008; Faraj et al., 2003; Whitson et al., 2007b; de Carvalho et al., 2009). To date, many clinical and preclinical studies, as well as in vitro analyses indicated an involvement of adiponectin in glucose regulation and fatty acid oxidation, thus an association between insulin sensitivity and circulating levels of adiponectin (Fruebis et al., 2001; Diez and Iglesias, 2003; Scherer et al., 2013; Yamauchi et al., 2013; Kadowaki et al., 2014). This suggests adiponection as a potential biomarker for insulin resistance (Scherer et al., 2013; Yamauchi et al., 2013; Kadowaki et al., 2014, Li et al., 2012).

Resistin

Resistin is a one of the family of cysteinerich resistin-like molecules (RELMs) produced by the adipocytes and the immune competent cells (Steppan et al., 2001a; Holcomb et al., 2000). It was discovered as a secreted product of murine adipose tissue and shown to positively correlate with body weight in animals and to be suppressed by antidiabetic drugs (i.e., thiazoledinedione) (Steppan et al., 2001b). Upon its discovery and regarding its link with inflammation, resistin also was termed FIZZ3 (found in inflammatory zone 3) related to a protein induced during lung inflammation known as 'found in inflammatory zone 1' (Holcomb et al., 2000). Resistin has been mostly studied in animals (Rabe et al., 2008; Won et al., 2009; Rajala et al., 2004; Singhal et al., 2007; Osawa et al., 2008) and is commonly associated with insulin mechanism: higher resistin was speculated to contribute to insulin resistance (Vendrell et al., 2004) and administration of exogenous resistin was found to result in impaired glucose tolerance and insulin resistance in mice (Steppan et al., 2001a).

Numerous studies suggested an association between increased serum resistin levels and obesity, as well as visceral fat (Degawa-Yamauchi et al., 2003; Matsuda et al., 2004; Vendrell et al., 2004; Pagano et al., 2005), insulin resistance (Malo et al., 2011) and inflammatory markers (Vendrell et al., 2004; Luis et al., 2010) in humans. In a study with children, significantly elevated resistin levels have been reported in children with metabolic syndrome compared to obese children without the metabolic syndrome or the healthy controls (Makni et al., 2013). However inconsistent results exist reporting lack of such correlations between resistin and body weight (Chen et al., 2005; Utzschneider et al., 2005; Won et al.,2009; Rabe et al.,2008; Koc et al., 2011) or insulin sensitivity (Pagano et al., 2005; Utzschneider et al., 2005).

The highest levels of murine resistin have been shown to be expressed in white adipose tissue (i.e., highest in the gonadal adipose tissue) (Steppan and Lazar, 2002). However, human resistin in adipose tissue is significantly lower and almost undetectable. It was shown to be expressed at the highest level in the bone marrow followed by the lung (Patel et al., 2003) with mRNA found in the nonfat cells of adipose depots (Fain et al., 2003) as well as in human placenta (Yura et al., 2003). The discrepancies between the reports may be due to the molecular and genetic diversity between human resistin with its murine counterpart (Steppan and Lazar, 2004). Thus, whether the physiology of mouse resistin is pertinent to humans needs to be determined.

Although there had been implications suggesting a possible role for resistin in the mechanism for the resolution of T2D following bariatric surgery, few studies investigated the alterations in resistin following RYGB in humans (Vendrell et al., 2004; Whitson et al., 2007b; Lee et al., 2011). One study showed no change in resistin levels in morbidly obese patients following gastric bypass at 6-month follow-up (Vendrell et al., 2004). However, they found that preoperative resistin levels were predictive of the extent of weight loss following RYGB (Vendrell et al., 2004). A study in nondiabetic RYGB patients showed a significant increase in resistin after 6 months following the surgery compared to the preoperative levels (Whitson et al., 2007b). However, the small sample size (n =4) weakens the results of this study. Furthermore, Lee et al. (2011) reported lower fasting plasma and postprandial (AUC following a 3-hour mixed meal tolerance test) resistin levels after 2 years following RYGB. Although there was not a preoperative baseline comparison, the intriguing aspect of this study was that they reported that the weight loss at the 2-year follow-up was similar between RYGB and sleeve gastrectomy patients however there was a significant difference in T2D remission in RYGB compared to the sleeve gastrectomy (81% vs. 19%). Thus the investigators suggested that resistin played a role in T2D resolution (Lee et al., 2011). Taken together, although a link between resistin and T2D has been reported, the normal physiologic role of resistin is still unclear, and the target tissues and molecular mechanisms by which resistin modulates glucose homeostasis require further investigation.

OTHER FACTORS RELATED TO GI TRACT

The alterations in the gut hormones caused by the re-arrangement of the gut leading restriction and malabsorption of the nutrients following RYGB have been long suggested to be the major factor behind the success of RYGB leading weight loss and T2D resolution (i.e the BRAVE effects of RYGB (Bile flow alterations, due to exclusion of the biliary limb, Reduced gastric size, Anatomic gut rearrangement, Vagal alterations secondary to the gut rearrangement, and Enteric (gut) hormone alterations). In addition to the BRAVE effects, recently, it has been suggested that the altered nutrient flux in the GI tract after RYGB might have different effects on the gut microbiota profile along the intestine. Accordingly, numerous studies have been conducted suggesting that the modulation of the gut microbial physiology to be responsible for the outcomes on energy homeostasis and metabolic function following RYGB (Erim et al., 2008, Papasavas et al., 2008). A few studies have examined the post-operative morphological changes following RYGB. Increased cell proliferation and downregulated apoptosis have been shown in the excluded gastric mucosa of the RYGB patents post-operatively compared to the non-operated obese controls (Safatle-Ribeiro et al., 2013). Such morphological and cellular alterations may be linked to changes in the number and function of enteroendocrine cells leading to increased plasma hormone levels after bariatric surgery.

CONCLUSION

Obesity is an epidemic and bariatric surgery is currently the most effective anti-obesity intervention and although the preference rate has been decreased, RYGB is still the most commonly performed bariatric surgery worldwide. However, the complete understanding of the mechanics behind the operation is still under investigation. It has been proposed that the anatomical re-arrangement alters food passage dynamics, evoking changes in gut hormone secretion to food that plays a major role in the efficacy of RYGB. During RYGB, a shortcut to the distal small intestine is created causing the bulk of foods passing into the small intestine without hindrance and aprolonged transit in the small intestine-is achieved (Dirksen et al., 2013b); the stomach and chyme are restricted, and excluded from the foregut making the operation both restrictive and malabsorptive in nature. Overall, anorexigenic GLP-1, PYY$_{3-36}$ (Ochner et al., 2011) and orexigenic ghrelin (Ybarra et al., 2009; Sundbom et al., 2007) have been the most intensively studied gut hormones following RYGB and are considered to be the best candidates for explaining the reductions in food intake and a consequent extensive weight loss. Caution must be always applied regarding the factors such as sample size, ethnicity, methodology (i.e., assay type, test meal load etc.) and obesity category, when interpreting the inconsistencies in findings regarding the gut hormone changes.Thus, contributions of reviews on the subject would prove to be very crucial for the field to have meaningful comparisons. Moreover, the physiological changes after RYGB are unlikely to be due to a single hormone, or single mechanism, but are more likely to due to the complex interplay between the gut hormones as well as the gut-brain communication that has not been reviewed here. Thus, new information is needed on the contribution of the different GI sites in reducing appetite and food intake in addition to its interactions with central systems on energy homeostasis and eating behavior. This will provide better understanding of the efficacy of RYGB on weight loss and may help to develop novel anti-obesity interventions to stimulate GI tract regions without surgery.

REFERENCES

Adams TD, Davidson LE, Litwin SE, et al. Health benefits of gastric bypass surgery after 6 years. *JAMA*. 2012;308(11):1122-1131.

Álvarez-Blasco F, Luque-Ramírez M, Escobar-Morreale HF. Obesity impairs general health-related quality of life (HR-QoL) in premenopausal women to a greater extent than polycystic ovary syndrome (PCOS). *Clinical endocrinology*. 2010;73(5):595-601.

Angrisani L, Santonicola A, Iovino P, Formisano G, Buchwald H, Scopinaro N. Bariatric surgery worldwide 2013. *Obesity surgery*. 2015 1;25(10):1822-32.

Arora S, Anubhuti. Role of neuropeptides in appetite regulation and obesity—review. *Neuropeptides*. 2006; 40:375–401.

Asakawa A, Inui A, Yuzuriha H, Ueno N, Katsuura G, Fujimiya M, Fujino MA, Niijima A, Meguid MM, Kasuga M. Characterization of the effects of pancreatic polypeptide in the regulation of energy balance. *Gastroenterology*. 2003;124(5):1325-36.

Ashby D, Bloom SR. Recent progress in PYY research—an update report for 8th NPY meeting. *Peptides*. 2007;28(2):198-202.

Ashrafian H, le Roux CW. Metabolic surgery and gut hormones–a review of bariatric entero-humoral modulation. *Physiology and behavior*. 2009;97(5):620-31.

Aynsley-Green A, Hussain K, Hall J, Saudubray JM, Nihoul-Fekete C, De Lonlay-Debeney P, Brunelle F, Otonkoski T, Thornton P, Lindley KJ. Practical management of hyperinsulinism in infancy. *Archives of Disease in Childhood-Fetal and Neonatal Edition*. 2000;82(2):F98-107.

Barkan AL, Dimaraki EV, Jessup SK, Symons KV, Ermolenko M, Jaffe CA. Ghrelin secretion in humans is sexually dimorphic, suppressed by somatostatin, and not affected by the ambient growth hormone levels. *The Journal of Clinical Endocrinology and Metabolism*. 2003;88(5):2180-4.

Bataille D, Gespach C, Tatemoto K, Marie JC, Coudray AM, Rosselin G, Mutt V. Bioactive enteroglucagon (oxyntomodulin): present knowledge on its chemical structure and its biological activities. *Peptides.* 1981 Dec 31;2:41-4.

Batterham RL, Cowley MA, Small CJ, Herzog H, Cohen MA, Dakin CL, Wren AM, Brynes AE, Low MJ, Ghatei MA, Cone RD and Bloom SR. Gut hormone PYY(3-36) physiologically inhibits food intake. *Nature,* 2002;418: 650-654.

Batterham RL, Cohen MA, Ellis SM, Le Roux CW, Withers DJ, Frost GS, Ghatei MA, Bloom SR. Inhibition of food intake in obese subjects by peptide YY3–36. *New England Journal of Medicine.* 2003a;349(10):941-8.

Batterham RL, Le Roux CW, Cohen MA, Park AJ, Ellis SM, Patterson M, Frost GS, Ghatei MA, Bloom SR. Pancreatic polypeptide reduces appetite and food intake in humans. *The Journal of Clinical Endocrinology and Metabolism.* 2003b; Aug 1;88(8):3989-92.

Beckman LM, Beckman TR, Sibley SD, Thomas W, Ikramuddin S, Kellogg TA, Ghatei MA, Bloom SR, le Roux CW, Earthman CP. Changes in gastrointestinal hormones and leptin after Roux-en-Y gastric bypass surgery. *Journal of Parenteral and Enteral Nutrition.* 2011 Mar 1;35(2):169-80.

Borai A, Livingstone C, Kaddam I, Ferns G. Selection of the appropriate method for the assessment of insulin resistance. *BMC medical research methodology.* 2011;11(1):1.

Borg CM, le Roux CW, Ghatei MA, Bloom SR, Patel AG, Aylwin SJ. Progressive rise in gut hormone levels after Roux-en-Y gastric bypass suggests gut adaptation and explains altered satiety. *Br J Surg.* 2006 Feb;93(2):210-5.

Bose M, Olivan B, Teixeira J, Pi-Sunyer FX, Laferrère B. Do Incretins play a role in the remission of type 2 diabetes after gastric bypass surgery: What are the evidence? *Obes Surg.* 2009; 19:217–229.

Bose M, Machineni S, Olivan B, Teixeira J, McGinty JJ, Bawa B, et al. Superior appetite hormone profile after equivalent weight loss by gastric bypass compared to gastric banding. *Obesity (Silver Spring).* 2010; 18:1085–1091.

Bryden MP, Ley RG, Sugarman JH. A left-ear advantage for identifying the emotional quality of tonal sequences. *Neuropsychologia.* 1982;20(1):83-7.

Buchwald H, Avidor Y, Braunwald E, Jensen MD, Pories W, Fahrbach K, Schoelles K. Bariatric surgery: a systematic review and meta-analysis. *JAMA* 2004;292(14):1724-37.

Buchwald H, Estok R, Fahrbach K et al. Weight and type 2 diabetes after bariatric surgery: systematic review and meta-analysis. *Am J Med* 2009a;122:248–256.e5.

Buchwald H, Oien DM. Metabolic/bariatric surgery worldwide 2008. *Obesity surgery*. 2009b;19(12):1605-11

Burrin DG, Petersen Y, Stoll B, Sangild P. Glucagon-like peptide 2: a nutrient-responsive gut growth factor. *The Journal of nutrition*. 2001;131(3):709-12.

Campos GM, Rabl C, Havel PJ, Rao M, Schwarz JM, Schambelan M, Mulligan K. Changes in post-prandial glucose and pancreatic hormones, and steady-state insulin and free fatty acids after gastric bypass surgery. *Surgery for Obesity and Related Diseases*. 2014 Feb 28;10(1):1-8.

Carlson JJ, Turpin AA, Wiebke G, Hunt SC, Adams TD. Pre- and post-prandial appetite hormone levels in normal weight and severely obese women. *Nutr Metab (Lond)*. 2009;6:32.

F. Carrasco, P. Rojas, A. Csendes et al., "Changes in ghrelin concentrations one year after resective and non-resective gastric bypass: associations with weight loss and energy and macronutrient intakes," *Nutrition*, 8(7)757–761, 2012.

Carroll JF, Kaiser KA, Franks SF, Deere C, Caffrey JL. Influence of BMI and gender on postprandial hormone responses. *Obesity* (Silver Spring). 2007 Dec;15(12):2974-83.

Carlson JJ, Turpin AA, Wiebke G, Hunt SC, Adams TD. Pre- and post-prandial appetite hormone levels in normal weight and severely obese women. *Nutr Metab (Lond)* 2009;6:32.

Carrasco F, Rojas P, Csendes A, Codoceo J, Inostroza J, Basfi-fer K, Papapietro K, Watkins G, Rojas J, Ruz M. Changes in ghrelin concentrations one year after resective and non-resective gastric bypass: associations with weight loss and energy and macronutrient intakes. *Nutrition*. 2012;28(7):757-61.

Carter ME, Soden ME, Zweifel LS, Palmiter RD. Genetic identification of a neural circuit that suppresses appetite. *Nature*. 2013;503(7474):111-4.

Cecil JE, Francis J, Read NW. Relative contributions of intestinal, gastric, oro-sensory influences and information to changes in appetite induced by the same liquid meal. *Appetite*. 1993;31(3):377-90.

Cheeseman CI, O'Neill D. Basolateral D-glucose transport activity along the crypt–villus axis in rat jejunum and upregulation induced by gastric inhibitory peptide and glucagon-like peptide-2. *Exp Physiol.* 1998;83:605–16.

Cheeseman CI, Tsang R. The effect of GIP and glucagon-like peptides on intestinal basolateral membrane hexose transport. *Am J Physiol.* 1996;271:G477–82.

Chen CC, Li TC, Li CI, Liu CS, Wang HJ, Lin CC. Serum resistin level among healthy subjects: relationship to anthropometric and metabolic parameters. *Metabolism.* 2005;54(4):471-5.

Choi K, Roh SG, Hong YH, Shrestha YB, Hishikawa D, Chen C, et al. The role of ghrelin and growth hormone secretagogues receptor on rat adipogenesis. *Endocrinology* 2003;144:754–9.

Chung J, Henry RR. Mechanisms of tumor-induced hypoglycemia with intra abdominal hemangiopericytoma. *J Clin Endocrinol Metab* 1996; 81: 919–925.

Cigdem Arica P, Kocael A, Tabak O, Taskin M, Zengin K, Uzun H. Plasma ghrelin, leptin, and orexin-A levels and insulin resistance after laparoscopic gastric band applications in morbidly obese patients. *Minerva Med* 2013;104(3):309e16.

Clements RH, Gonzalez QH, Long CI, et al. Hormonal changes after Roux-en Y gastric bypass for morbid obesity and the control of type-II diabetes mellitus. *Am Surg.* 2004;70:1–4.

Cohen MA, Ellis SM, Le Roux CW, Batterham RL, Park A, Patterson M, Frost GS, Ghatei MA, Bloom SR. Oxyntomodulin suppresses appetite and reduces food intake in humans. *J Clin Endocrinol Metab* 2003; 88:4696–4701.

Cohen RV, Schiavon CA, Pinheiro JS, Correa JL, Rubino F. Duodenal-jejunal bypass for the treatment of type 2 diabetes in patients with body mass index of 22–34 kg/m2: a report of 2 cases. *Surg Obes Relat Dis* 2007; 3(2): 195–197.

Considine RV, Sinha MK, Heiman ML, Kriauciunas A, Stephens TW, Nyce MR, Ohannesian JP, Marco CC, McKee LJ, Bauer TL, Caro JF. Serum immunoreactive-leptin concentrations in normal-weight and obese humans. *New England Journal of Medicine.* 1996;334(5):292-5.

Corp ES, Woods SC, Porte D, Dorsa DM, Figlewicz DP, Baskin DG. Localization of 125I-insulin binding sites in the rat hypothalamus by quantitative autoradiography. *Neuroscience letters.* 1986;70(1):17-22.

Corp ES, McQuade J, Moran TH and Smith GP. Characterization of type A and type B CCK receptor binding sites in rat vagus nerve. *Brain Res,* 1993; 623: 161-166.

Cox HM. Neuropeptide Y receptors; antisecretory control of intestinal epithelial function. *Auton. Neurosci.* 2007;133, 76–85.

Cremonini F, Camilleri M, Gonenne J, Stephens D, Oenning L, Baxter K, Foxx-Orenstein A, Burton D. Effect of somatostatin analog on postprandial satiation in obesity. *Obesity research.* 2005;13(9):1572-9.

Cummings DE, Purnell JQ, Frayo RS, Schmidova K, Wisse BE, Weigle DS. A preprandial rise in plasma ghrelin levels suggests a role in meal initiation in humans. *Diabetes* 2001;50:1714–9.

Cummings DE, Weigle DS, Frayo RS, et al. Plasma ghrelin levels after diet-induced weight loss or gastric bypass surgery. *N Engl J Med.* 2002;346:1623–30.

Creutzfeldt W. The entero-insular axis in type 2 diabetes— incretins as therapeutic agents. *Exp Clin Endocrinol Diabetes.* 2001;109(2):288–303.

Cummings DE, Overduin J, Foster-Schubert KE. Gastric bypass for obesity: mechanisms of weight loss and diabetes resolution. *The journal of clinical endocrinology and metabolism.* 2004;89(6):2608-15.

Dakin CL, Gunn I, Small CJ, Edwards CM, Hay DL, Smith DM, Ghatei MA, Bloom SR. Oxyntomodulin inhibits food intake in the rat. *Endocrinology.* 2001;142(10):4244-50.

de Carvalho CP, Marin DM, de Souza AL, Pareja JC, Chaim EA, de Barros Mazon S, et al. GLP-1 and adiponectin: effect of weight loss after dietary restriction and gastric bypass in morbidly obese patients with normal and abnormal glucose metabolism. *Obes Surg.* 2009;19:313–320.

Degawa-Yamauchi M, Bovenkerk JE, Juliar BE, Watson W, Kerr K, Jones R, Zhu Q, Considine RV Serum resistin (FIZZ3) protein is increased in obese humans. *J Clin Endocrinol Metab* 2003; 88:5452–5455.

de Hollanda A, Jiménez A, Corcelles R, Lacy AM, Patrascioiu I, Vidal J. Gastrointestinal hormones and weight loss response after Roux-en-Y gastric bypass. *Surgery for Obesity and Related Diseases.* 2014;10(5):814-9.

De León DD, Crutchlow MF, Ham JY, Stoffers DA. Role of glucagon-like peptide-1 in the pathogenesis and treatment of diabetes mellitus. *Int J Biochem Cell Biol* 2006;38:845–859.

De Luis DA, Gonzalez Sagrado M, Conde R, Aller R, Izaola O. Resistin levels and inflammatory markers in patients with morbid obesity. *Nutr Hosp.* 2010;25(4):630-4.

DePaula AL, Macedo AL, Schraibman V, Mota BR, Vencio S. Hormonal evaluation following laparoscopic treatment of type 2 diabetes mellitus patients with BMI 20-34. *Surg Endosc.* 2009 Aug;23(8):1724-32.

Despres JP, Lemieux I. Abdominal obesity and metabolic syndrome. *Nature* 2006;444:881–887.

Diez JJ and Iglesias P. The role of the novel adipocyte-derived hormone adiponectin in human disease. *Eur J Endocrinol,* 2003; 148: 293-300.

Dirksen C, Hansen DL, Madsbad S, Hvolris LE, Naver LS, Holst JJ, Worm D. Postprandial diabetic glucose tolerance is normalized by gastric bypass feeding as opposed to gastric feeding and is associated with exaggerated GLP-1 secretion: a case report. *Diabetes Care* 2010; 33(2): 375–377.

Dirksen C, Jørgensen NB, Bojsen-Møller, KN, Kielgast U, Jacobsen SH, Clausen TR, et al. Gut hormones, early dumping and resting energy expenditure in patients with good and poor weight loss response after Roux-en-Y gastric bypass. *International journal of obesity* 2013a, 37(11),1452-9.

Dirksen C, Damgaard M, Bojsen-Møller KN, Jørgensen NB, Kielgast U, Jacobsen SH, Naver LS, Worm D, Holst JJ, Madsbad S, Hansen DL. Fast pouch emptying, delayed small intestinal transit, and exaggerated gut hormone responses after Roux-en-Y gastric bypass. *Neurogastroenterology and Motility.* 2013b;25(4):346-e255.

Doyle ME, Egan JM. Mechanisms of action of glucagon-like peptide 1 in the pancreas. *Pharmacol Ther* 2007;113:546–593.

Dunning BE, Gerich JE. The role of alpha-cell dysregulation in fasting and postprandial hyperglycemia in type 2 diabetes and therapeutic implications. *Endocr Rev* 2007; 28:253–283.

Edholm D, Svensson F, Naslund I, Karlsson FA, Rask E, Sundbom M. Long-term results 11 years after primary gastric bypass in 384 patients. *Surg Obes Relat Dis* 2013;9:708.

Edwards C, Hindle AK, Fu S, Brody F. Downregulation of leptin and resistin expression in blood following bariatric surgery. *Surg Endosc* 2011; 25:1962–1968.

Ekblad E, Sundler F, Distribution of pancreatic polypeptide and peptide YY. *Peptides* 2002; 23, 251–261.

English PJ, Ghatei MA, Malik IA, Bloom SR, Wilding JP. Food fails to suppress ghrelin levels in obese humans. *J Clin Endocrinol Metab* 2002;87:2984.

Erim T, Cruz-Correa MR, Szomstein S, Velis E, and Rosenthal R. Prevalence of Helicobacter pylori seropositivity among patients undergoing bariatric surgery: a preliminary study. *World journal of surgery.* 2008; 32(9): 2021-2025.

Fain JN, Cheema PS, Bahouth SW, Lloyd Hiler M. Resistin release by human adipose tissue explants in primary culture. *Biochem Biophys Res Commun* 2003; 300: 674–8.

Falkén Y, Hellström PM, Holst JJ, Nälund E. Changes in glucose homeostasis after Roux-en-Y gastric bypass surgery for obesity at day three, two months, and one year after surgery: role of gut peptides. *J Clin Endocrinol Metab* 2011;96:2227-2235.

Faraj M, Havel PJ, Phelis S, Blank D, Sniderman AD, Cianflone K. Plasma acylation-stimulating protein, adiponectin, leptin, and ghrelin before and after weight loss induced by gastric bypass surgery in morbidly obese subjects. *J Clin Endocrinol Metab.* 2003; 88:1594–1602.

Feinle C, O'Donovan D, Doran S, Andrews JM, Wishart J, Chapman I and Horowitz M. Effects of fat digestion on appetite, APD motility, and gut hormones in response to duodenal fat infusion in humans. *Am J Physiol Gastrointest Liver Physiol,* 2003; 284: G798-807.

Ferrannini E, Mingrone G. Impact of different bariatric surgical procedures on insulin action and beta-cell function in type 2 diabetes. *Diabetes Care* 2009;32:514-20.

Field BC, Chaudhri OB, Bloom SR. Bowels control brain: gut hormones and obesity. *Nature reviews endocrinology.* 2010;6(8):444-53.

Fiocca R, Sessa F, Tenti P, Usellini L, Capella C, O'Hare M.M, Solcia E. Pancreatic Polypeptide (PP) cells in the PP-rich lobe of the human pancreas are indentified ultrastructurally and immunocytochemically as F cells. *Histochemistry* 1983; 77: 511-523.

Flegal, K.M. and D.F. Williamson, Incident CHD and excess body weight in the US population. *Obesity (Silver Spring),* 2010. 18(6): 1069; author reply 1069-70.

Foschi D, Corsi F, Colombo F, Vago T, Bevilaqua M, Rizzi A, et al. Different effects of vertical banded gastroplasty and Roux-en-Y gastric bypass on meal inhibition of ghrelin secretion in morbidly obese patients. *J Invest Surg* 2008;21:77–81.

Fruebis J, Tsao TS, Javorschi S, Ebbets-Reed D, Erickson MR, Yen FT, Bihain BE, Lodish HF. Proteolytic cleavage product of 30-kDa adipocyte complement-related protein increases fatty acid oxidation in muscle and causes weight loss in mice. *Proceedings of the national academy of sciences.* 2001;98(4):2005-10.

Frühbeck G, Diez-Caballero A, G_omez-Ambrosi J, Gil MJ, Monreal I, Salvador J, et al. Disruption of the leptin-insulin relationship in obesemen24 hours after laparoscopic adjustable silicone gastric banding. *Obes Surg* 2002;12(3):366e71.

Frühbeck G, Rotellar F, Hernandez-Lizoain JL, Gil MJ, Gomez-Ambrosi J, Salvador J, et al. Fasting plasma ghrelin concentrations 6 months after gastric bypass are not determined by weight loss or changes in insulinemia. *Obes Surg* 2004;14:1208–15.

Gaitonde S, Kohli R, Seeley R. The role of the gut hormone GLP-1 in the metabolic improvements caused by ileal transposition. *J Surg Res* 2012; 178(1): 33–39.

Garcia de la Torre N, Rubio MA, Bordiu E, Cabrerizo L, Aparicio E, Hernandez C, et al. Effects of weight loss after bariatric surgery for morbid obesity on vascular endothelial growth factor-A, adipocytokines, and insulin. *J Clin Endocrinol Metab* 2008;93: 4276–81.

Garcia-Fuentes E, Garrido-Sanchez L, Garcia-Almeida JM, Garcia-Arnes J, Gallego-Perales JL, Rivas-Marin J, Morcillo S, Cardona I, Soriguer F. Different effect of laparoscopic Roux-en-Y gastric bypass and open biliopancreatic diversion of Scopinaro on serum PYY and ghrelin levels. *Obesity surgery*. 2008;18(11):1424-9.

Gautier JF, Choukem SP, Girard J. Physiology of incretins (GIP and GLP-1) and abnormalities in type 2 diabetes. *Diabetes Metab* 2008;34(2):S65–S72.

Geary N, Kissileff HR, Pi-Sunyer FX, Hinton VE. Individual, but not simultaneous, glucagon and cholecystokinin infusions inhibit feeding in men. *American journal of physiology-regulatory, integrative and comparative physiology*. 1992;262(6):R975-80.

Ghatei MA, Uttenthal LO, Christofides ND, Bryant MG, Bloom SR. Molecular Forms of Human Enteroglucagon in Tissue and Plasma: Plasma Responses to Nutrient Stimuli in Health and in Disorders of the Upper Gastrointestinal Tract*. *The journal of clinical endocrinology and metabolism. 1983*;57(3):488-95.

Gibbs J, Young RC and Smith GP. Cholecystokinin decreases food intake in rats. *J Comp Physiol Psychol*, 1973;84: 488-495.

Gloy VL, Briel M, Bhatt DL, Kashyap SR, Schauer PR, Mingrone G, et al. Bariatric surgery versus non-surgical treatment for obesity: a systematic review and meta-analysis of randomised controlled trials. *British Medical Journal*, 2013;347, f5934.

Goldfine AB, Mun EC, Devine E, Bernier R, Baz-Hecht M, Jones DB, et al. Patients with neuroglycopenia after gastric bypass surgery have exaggerated incretin and insulin secretory responses to a mixed meal. *J Clin Endocrinol Metab* 2007; 92(12): 4678–4685.

Goldstein JM, Jerram M, Poldrack R, Ahern T, Kennedy DN, Seidman LJ, et al. Hormonal cycle modulates arousal circuitry in women using functional magnetic resonance imaging. *J Neurosci.* 2005;25(40):9309-16.

Gortmaker, S.L., et al., Social and economic consequences of overweight in adolescence and young adulthood. *N Engl J Med,* 1993. 329(14): p. 1008-12.

Gourcerol G, Coskun T, Craft LS, Mayer JP, Heiman ML, Wang L, Million M, St-Pierre DH, Taché Y. Preproghrelin-derived peptide, obestatin, fails to influence food intake in lean or obese rodents. *Obesity.* 2007;15(11):2643-52.

Grong E, Græslie H, Munkvold B, Arbo IB, Kulseng BE, Waldum HL, Mårvik R. Gastrin secretion after bariatric surgery—response to a protein-rich mixed meal following Roux-En-Y gastric bypass and sleeve gastrectomy: a pilot study in normoglycemic women. *Obesity surgery.* 2015;27:1-9.

Gunstad J, Strain G, Devlin MJ, Wing R, Cohen RA, Paul RH et al. Improved memory function 12 weeks after bariatric surgery. *Surg Obes Relat Dis* 2011; 7: 465–472.

Guo Y, Ma L, Enriori PJ, Koska J, Franks PW, Brookshire T, Cowley MA, Salbe AD, DelParigi A, Tataranni PA. Physiological evidence for the involvement of peptide YY in the regulation of energy homeostasis in humans. *Obesity.* 2006;14(9):1562-70.

Guo ZF, Zheng X, Qin Y-W, et al. Circulating preprandial ghrelin to obestatin ratio is increased in human obesity. *J Clin Endocrinol Metab.* 2007;92:1875–80.

Herrmann, C., et al., Glucagon-like peptide-1 and glucose-dependent insulin-releasing polypeptide plasma levels in response to nutrients. *Digestion,* 1995;56(2):117-26.

Holcomb IN, Kabakoff RC, Chan B et al. FIZZ1, a novel cysteine- rich secreted protein associated with pulmonary inflammation, defines a new gene family. *EMBO J* 2000; 19: 4046–55.

Holdstock C, Engstrom BE, Ohrvall M, Lind L, Sundbom M, Karlsson FA. Ghrelin and adipose tissue regulatory peptides: effect of gastric bypass surgery in obese humans. *J Clin Endocrinol Metab.* 2003;88:3177–83.

Holdstock C, Zethelius B, Sundbom M, Karlsson FA, Edén Engström B. Postprandial changes in gut regulatory peptides in gastric bypass patients. *Int J Obes (Lond)* 2008; 32(11): 1640–1646.

Holst JJ, Pedersen JH, Baldissera F, Stadil F. Circulating glucagon after total pancreatectomy in man. *Diabetologia* 1983; 25:396–399.

Holst JJ. Glucagon and glucagon-like peptides 1 and 2. Cellular Peptide Hormone Synthesis and Secretory Pathways. Berlin Heidelberg. *Springer.* 2009.

Holzer HH, Turkelson CM, Solomon TE and Raybould HE. Intestinal lipid inhibits gastric emptying via CCK and a vagal capsaicin-sensitive afferent pathway in rats. *Am J Physiol,* 1994;267: G625-629.

Howard AD, Feighner SD, Cully DF, Arena JP, Liberator PA, Rosenblum CI, et al. A receptor in pituitary and hypothalamus that functions in growth hormone release. *Science* 1996;273:974–7.

Huda MS, Durham BH, Wong SP, Deepak D, Kerrigan D, McCulloch P, Ranganath L, Pinkney J, Wilding JP. Plasma obestatin levels are lower in obese and post-gastrectomy subjects, but do not change in response to a meal. *International journal of obesity.* 2008;32(1):129-35.

Itoh H, Takei K. Immunohistochemical and statistical studies on the islets of Langerhans pancreas in autopsied patients after gastrectomy. *Human pathology.* 2000;31(11):1368-76.

Jacobsen SH, Olesen SC, Dirksen C, Jørgensen NB, Bojsen-Møller KN, Kielgast U, Worm D, Almdal T, Naver LS, Hvolris LE, Rehfeld JF. Changes in gastrointestinal hormone responses, insulin sensitivity, and beta-cell function within 2 weeks after gastric bypass in non-diabetic subjects. *Obesity surgery.* 2012;22(7):1084-96.

Jang HJ, Kokrashvili Z, Theodorakis MJ, Carlson OD, Kim BJ, Zhou J, Kim HH, Xu X, Chan SL, Juhaszova M, et al. Gut-expressed gustducin and taste receptors regulate secretion of glucagon-like peptide-1. *Proc Natl Acad Sci USA* 2007;104:15069–15074.

Jensen DE, Nguo K, Baxter KA, Cardinal JW, King NA, Ware RS, Truby H, Batch JA. Fasting gut hormone levels change with modest weight loss in obese adolescents. *Pediatric obesity.* 2015;10(5):380-7.

Kadowaki T, Yamauchi T, Okada-Iwabu M, Iwabu M. Adiponectin and its receptors: implications for obesity-associated diseases and longevity. *Lancet Diabetes Endocrinol.* 2014;2(1):8-9.

Kahn SE, D'Alessio DA, Schwartz MW, Fujimoto WY, Ensinck JW, Taborsky GJ, Porte D. Evidence of cosecretion of islet amyloid polypeptide and insulin by β-cells. *Diabetes.* 1990;39(5):634-8.

Kahn SE, Cooper ME, Del Prato S. Pathophysiology and treatment of type 2 diabetes: perspectives on the past, present, and future. *Lancet.* 2014;383(9922):1068-83.

Kalogeris TJ, Reidelberger RD, Mendel VE. Effect of nutrient density and composition of liquid meals on gastric emptying in feeding rats. *American journal of physiology-regulatory, integrative and comparative physiology.* 1983;244(6):R865-71.

Karra E, Chandarana K, Batterham RL. The role of peptide YY in appetite regulation and obesity. *The journal of physiology.* 2009;587(1):19-25.

Karamanakos SN, Vagenas K, Kalfarentzos F, Alexandrides TK. Weight loss, appetite suppression, and changes in fasting and postprandial ghrelin and peptide-YY levels after Roux-en- Y gastric bypass and sleeve gastrectomy: a prospective, double blind study. *Ann Surg.* 2008;247:401–407.

Katsusuke S, Takeuchi T, Watanabe S, Nishiwaki H. Postprandial plasma cholecystokinin response in patients after gastrectomy and pancreatoduodenectomy. *Am J Gastroenterol.* 2008; 81:1038–1042.

Kellum JM, Kuemmerle JF, O'Dorisio TM, Rayford P, Martin D, Engle K, et al. Gastrointestinal hormone responses to meals before and after gastric bypass and vertical banded gastroplasty. *Ann Surg.*1990;211:763–770.

Kissileff HR, Pi-Sunyer FX, Thornton J and Smith GP. C-terminal octapeptide of cholecystokinin decreases food intake in man. *Am J Clin Nutr,* 1981;34: 154-160.

Kissileff HR, Carretta JC, Geliebter A and Pi-Sunyer FX. Cholecystokinin and stomach distension combine to reduce food intake in humans. *Am j physiol regul integr comp physiol,* 2003; 285: R992-998.

Kloting N, Graham TE, Berndt J, et al. Serum retinol-binding protein is more high-ly expressed in visceral than in subcutaneous adipose tissue and is a marker of intra-abdominal obesity fat mass. *Cell Metab* 2007;6:79–87.

Knerr I, Herzog D, Rauh M, RascherW, Horbach T. Leptin and ghrelin expression in adipose tissues and serum levels in gastric banding patients. *Eur J Clin Invest* 2006;36(6):389e94.

Koç F, Tokaç M, Kocabas V, Kaya C, Buyukbas S, Erdem S, Karabag T, Demir K, Alihanoglu Y, Kaya A. Ghrelin, resistin and leptin levels in patients with metabolic syndrome. *European Journal of General Medicine. Eur J Gen Med,* 2011;8 (2) 92–97.

Kojima M, Hosoda H, Date Y, Nakazato M, Matsuo H, Kangawa K. Ghrelin is a growth-hormone-releasing acylated peptide from stomach. *Nature* 1999;402: 656–60.

Komatsu R, Matsuyama T, Namba M, Watanabe N, Itoh H, Kono N, Tarui S. Glucagonostatic and insulinotropic action of glucagonlike peptide I-(7–36)-amide. *Diabetes* 1989;38:902–905.

Korner J, Inabnet W, Conwell IM, Taveras C, Daud A, Olivero- Rivera L, Restuccia NL, Bessler M. Differential effects of gastric bypass and banding on circulating gut hormone and leptin levels. *Obesity (Silver Spring)* 2006; 14(9): 1553–1561.

Korner J, Bessler M, Inabnet W, Taveras C, Holst JJ. Exaggerated glucagon-like peptide-1 and blunted glucose-dependent insulinotropic peptide secretion are associated with Roux-en-Y gastric bypass but not adjustable gastric banding. *Surg Obes Relat Dis* 2007; 3(6): 597–601.

Korner J, Inabnet W, Febres G, Conwell IM, McMahon DJ, Salas R, et al. Prospective study of gut hormone and metabolic changes after adjustable gastric banding and Roux-en-Y gastric bypass. *Int J Obes (Lond).* 2009 Jul;33(7):786-95.

Kotidis EV, Koliakos GG, Baltzopoulos VG, Ioannidis KN, Yovos JG, Papavramidis ST. Serum ghrelin, leptin and adiponectin levels before and after weight loss: comparison of three methods of treatment—prospective study. *Obes Surg.* 2006; 16:1425–1432.

Lacquaniti A, Donato V, Chirico V, Buemi A, Buemi M. Obestatin: an interesting but controversial gut hormone. *Annals of nutrition and metabolism.* 2011;59(2-4):193-9.

Laferrere B, Heshka S, Wang K, et al. Incretin levels and effect are markedly enhanced 1 month after Roux-en-Y gastric bypass surgery in obese patients with type 2 diabetes. *Diabetes Care* 2007; 30:1709–16.

Laferrère B, Teixeira J, McGinty J, Tran H, Egger JR, Colarusso A, et al. Effect of weight loss by gastric bypass surgery versus hypocaloric diet on glucose and incretin levels in patients with type 2 diabetes. *J Clin Endocrinol Metab* 2008; 93(7): 2479–2485.

Laferrere B, Swerdlow N, Bawa B, Arias S, Bose M, Olivan B, Teixeira J, McGinty J, Rother KI. Rise of oxyntomodulin in response to oral glucose after gastric bypass surgery in patients with type 2 diabetes. *The journal of clinical endocrinology and metabolism.* 2010;95(8):4072-6.

Lal S, McLaughlin J, Barlow J, D'Amato M, Giacovelli G, Varro A, Dockray GJ and Thompson DG. Cholecystokinin pathways modulate sensations induced by gastric distension in humans. *Am j physiol gastrointest liver physiol,* 2004; 287: G72-79.

Lee WJ, Chen CY, Chong K, et al. Changes in postprandial gut hormones after metabolic surgery: a comparison of gastric bypass and sleeve gastrectomy. *Surg Obes Relat Dis.* 2011;7(6) 683–90.

le Roux CW, Aylwin SJ, Batterham RL, Borg CM, Coyle F, Prasad V, et al. Gut hormone profiles following bariatric surgery favor an anorectic state, facilitate weight loss, and improve metabolic parameters. *Ann Surg.* 2006;243(1):108-14.

le Roux CW, Welbourn R, Werling M, Osborne A, Kokkinos A, Laurenius A, et al. Gut hormones as mediators of appetite and weight loss after Roux-en-Y gastric bypass. *Ann Surg.* 2007; 246:780–785.

le Roux CW, Borg C, Wallis K, Vincent RP, Bueter M, Goodlad R, Ghatei MA, Patel A, Bloom SR, Aylwin SJ. Gut hypertrophy after gastric bypass is associated with increased glucagon-like peptide 2 and intestinal crypt cell proliferation. *Annals of surgery.* 2010;252(1):50-6.

Li FY, Lam KS, Xu A. Therapeutic perspectives for adiponectin: an update. *Current medicinal chemistry.* 2012;19(32):5513-23.

Liddle RA, Goldfine ID, Rosen MS, Taplitz RA and Williams JA. Cholecystokinin bioactivity in human plasma. Molecular forms, responses to feeding, and relationship to gallbladder contraction. *J Clin Invest,* 1985;75: 1144-1152.

Lieverse RJ, Jansen JB, Masclee AM and Lamers CB. Satiety effects of cholecystokinin in humans. *Gastroenterology,* 1994;106: 1451-1454.

Lin E, Gletsu N, Fugate K, McClusky D, Gu LH, Zhu JL, et al. The effects of gastric surgery on systemic ghrelin levels in the morbidly obese. *Arch Surg* 2004;139:780–4.

Lippl F, Erdmann J, Lichter N, et al. Relation of plasma obestatin levels to BMI, gender, age and insulin. *Horm Metab Res.* 2008;40:806–12.

Lutter M and Nestler EJ. Homeostatic and hedonic signals interact in the regulation of food intake. *J Nutr,* 2009;139(3):629-32.

Lutz TA. Pancreatic amylin as a centrally acting satiating hormone. *Curr Drug Targets* 2005; 6: 181–189.

Lutz TA, Meyer U. Amylin at the interface between metabolic and neurodegenerative disorders. *Frontiers in neuroscience.* 2015; 9:216.

Maida A, Lovshin JA, Baggio LL, Drucker DJ. The glucagon-like peptide-1 receptor agonist oxyntomodulin enhances β-cell function but does not inhibit gastric emptying in mice. *Endocrinology* 2008;149:5670–5678.

Makni E, Moalla W, Benezzeddine-Boussaidi L, Lac G, Tabka Z, Elloumi M. Correlation of resistin with inflammatory and cardiometabolic markers in obese adolescents with and without metabolic syndrome. *Obes Facts* 2013;6(4):393–404.

Malo E, Ukkola O, Jokela M, et al: Resistin is an indicator of the metabolic syndrome according to five different definitions in the Finnish health 2000 survey. *Metab Syndr Relat Disord* 2011;9:203-210.

Martin JR, Novin D. Decreased feeding in rats following hepatic-portal infusion of glucagon. *Physiology and behavior.* 1977;19(4):461-6.

Martins C, Kjelstrup L, Mostad IL, Kulseng B. Impact of sustained weight loss achieved through Roux-en-Y gastric bypass or a lifestyle intervention on ghrelin, obestatin, and ghrelin/obestatin ratio in morbidly obese patients. *Obesity surgery.* 2011;21(6):751-8.

Mason EE. Ilial transposition and enteroglucagon/GLP-1 in obesity (and diabetic?) surgery. *Obes Surg* 1999; 9(3): 223–228.

Matikainen N, Björnson E, Söderlund S, Borén C, Eliasson B, Pietiläinen KH, Bogl LH, Hakkarainen A, Lundbom N, Rivellese A, Riccardi G. Minor Contribution of Endogenous GLP-1 and GLP-2 to Postprandial Lipemia in Obese Men. *PloS one.* 2016;11(1).

Matsuda M, Kawasaki F, Yamada K, Kanda Y, Saito M, Eto M, et al. Impact of adiposity and plasma adipocytokines on diabetic angiopathies in Japanese type 2 diabetic subjects. *Diabet Med* 2004;21(8):881–8.

McIntosh CH, Widenmaier S, Kim SJ. Glucose-dependent insulinotropic polypeptide (gastric inhibitory polypeptide; GIP). *Horm.* 2009;80:409–71.

McLaughlin J, Lucà MG, Jones MN, D'Amato M, Dockray GJ, Thompson DG. Fatty acid chain length determines cholecystokinin secretion and effect on human gastric motility. *Gastroenterology.* 1999;116(1):46-53.

Meguid MM, Glade MJ, Middleton FA. Weight regain after Roux-en-Y: a significant 20% complication related to PYY. *Nutrition.* 2008;24(9):832-42.

Mei N, Intestinal chemosensitivity. *Physiol Rev,* 1985;65(2):211-37.

Menéndez J, Atrens DM. Insulin and the paraventricular hypothalamus: modulation of energy balance. *Brain research.* 1991;555(2):193-201.

Michel MC, Beck-Sickinger A, Cox H, Doods HN, Herzog H, Larhammar D, Quirion R, Schwartz T, Westfall T. XVI. International Union of Pharmacology recommendations for the nomenclature of neuropeptide Y, peptide YY, and pancreatic polypeptide receptors. *Pharmacological reviews.* 1998;50(1):143-50.

Misra M, Miller KK, Tsai P, Gallagher K, Lin A, Lee N, Herzog DB, Klibanski A. Elevated peptide YY levels in adolescent girls with anorexia nervosa. *The journal of clinical endocrinology and metabolism.* 2006;91(3):1027-33.

Molina A, Vendrell J, Gutiérrez C, Simón I, Masdevall C, Soler J, Gómez JM. Insulin resistance, leptin and TNF-α system in morbidly obese women after gastric bypass. *Obesity surgery.* 2003;13(4):615-21.

Mollet A, Meier S, Grabler V, Gilg S, Scharrer E, and Lutz TA. Endogenous amylin contributes to the anorectic effects of cholecystokinin and bombesin. *Peptides* 2003a; 24:91–98.

Moran TH, Kornbluh R, Moore K and Schwartz GJ. Cholecystokinin inhibits gastric emptying and contracts the pyloric sphincter in rats by interacting with low affinity CCK receptor sites. 1994; *Regul Pept*, 52: 165-172.

Moran TH. Cholecystokinin and satiety: current perspectives. *Nutrition.* 2000;16:858–65.

Moran-Atkin E, Brody F, Fu SW, Rojkind M. Changes in GIP gene expression following bariatric surgery. *Surg Endosc*, 2013;27:2492–2497.

Moriarty P, Dimaline R, Thompson DG and Dockray GJ. Characterization of cholecystokinin A and cholecystokinin B receptors expressed by vagal afferent neurons. *Neuroscience,* 1997;79: 905-913.

Morinigo R, Casamitjana R, Moize V, Lacy AM, Delgado S, Gomis R, et al. Short-term effects of gastric bypass surgery on circulating ghrelin levels. *Obes Res* 2004;12: 1108–16.

Morinigo R, Moize V, Musri M, Lacy AM, Navarro S, Marin JL, et al. Glucagon-like peptide-1, peptide YY, hunger, and satiety after gastric bypass surgery in morbidly obese subjects. *J Clin Endocrinol Metab.* 2006; 91:1735–1740.

Morinigo R, Vidal J, Lacy AM, Delgado S, Casamitjana R, Gomis R. Circulating peptide YY, weight loss, and glucose homeostasis after gastric bypass surgery in morbidly obese subjects. *Ann Surg.* 2008; 247:270–275.

Nannipieri M, Baldi S, Mari A, Colligiani D, Guarino D, Camastra S, Barsotti E, Berta R, Moriconi D, Bellini R, Anselmino M. Roux-en-Y gastric bypass and sleeve gastrectomy: mechanisms of diabetes remission and role of gut hormones. *The journal of clinical endocrinology and metabolism.* 2013;98(11):4391-9.

Näslund E, King N, Mansten S, Adner N, Holst JJ, Gutniak M, Hellström PM. Prandial subcutaneous injections of glucagon-like peptide-1 cause weight loss in obese human subjects. *British journal of nutrition.* 2004;91(03):439-46.

Naslund E, Hellstrom PM. Appetite signaling: from gut peptides and enteric nerves to brain. *Physiol Behav.* 2007;92(1-2):256-62.

Nauck MA, Homberger E, Siegel EG, Allen RC, Eaton RP, Ebert R, Creutzfeldt W. Incretin effects of increasing glucose loads in man calculated from venous insulin and C-peptide responses. *J Clin Endocrinol Metab* 1986; 63:492–498.

Nijhuis J, van Dielen FM, Buurman WA, Greve JW. Ghrelin, leptin and insulin levels after restrictive surgery: a 2-year follow-up study. *Obes Surg.* 2004;14(6):783-7.

Ochner CN, Stice E, Hutchins E, Afifi L, Geliebter A, Hirsch J, Teixeira J. Relation between changes in neural responsivity and reductions in desire to eat high-calorie foods following gastric bypass surgery. *Neuroscience.* 2012;209:128-35.

Osawa H, Ochi M, Tabara Y, Kato K, Yamauchi J, Takata Y, et al. Serum resistin is positively correlated with the accumulation of metabolic syndrome factors in type 2 diabetes. *Clin Endocrinol (Oxf).* 2008; 69:74–80.

Pagano C, Marin O, Calcagno A, Schiappelli P, Pilon C, Milan G, et al. Increased serum resistin in adults with Prader-Willi syndrome is related to obesity and not to insulin resistance. *J Clin Endocrinol Metab 2005*;90(7):4335–40.

Papasavas PK, Gagné DJ, Donnelly PE, Salgado J, Urbandt JE, Burton KK, et al. Prevalence of Helicobacter pylori infection and value of preoperative testing and treatment in patients undergoing laparoscopic Roux-en-Y gastric bypass. *Surgery for obesity and related diseases.* 2008; 4(3): 383-388.

Pardina E, Lopez-Tejero MD, Llamas R, Catalan R, Galard R, Allende H, et al. Ghrelin and apolipoprotein AIV levels show opposite trends to leptin levels during weight loss in morbidly obese patients. *Obes Surg* 2009;19:1414–23.

Parker BA, Doran S, Wishart J, Horowitz M and Chapman IM. Effects of small intestinal and gastric glucose administration on the suppression of plasma ghrelin concentrations in healthy older men and women. *Clin Endocrinol (Oxf),* 2005; 62: 539-546.

Paschetta E, Hvalryg M, Musso G. Glucose-dependent insulinotropic polypeptide: from pathophysiology to therapeutic opportunities in obesity-associated disorders. *Obesity Reviews.* 2011;12(10):813-28.

Patel L, Buckels AC, Kinghorn IJ, Murdock PR, Holbrook JD, Plumpton C, Macphee CH, Smith SA. Resistin is expressed in human macrophages and directly regulated by PPARγ activators. *Biochemical and biophysical research communications.* 2003;300(2):472-6.

Penick SB, Hinkle Jr LE, Paulsen EG. Depression of food intake induced in healthy subjects by glucagon. *New england journal of medicine.* 1961;264(18):893-7.

Peterli R, Wolnerhanssen B, Peters T, Devaux N, Kern B, Christoffel-Courtin C, et al. Improvement in glucose metabolism after bariatric surgery: comparison of laparoscopic Roux-en-Y gastric bypass and laparoscopic sleeve gastrectomy: a prospective randomized trial. *Ann Surg.* 2009; 250:234–241.

Peterli R, Steinert RE, Woelnerhanssen B, Peters T, Christoffel-Courtin C, Gass M, Kern B, von Fluee M, Beginger C. Metabolic and hormonal changes after laparoscopic Roux-en-Y gastric bypass and sleeve gastrectomy: a randomized, prospective trial. *Obes Surg.* 2012;22(5):740-8.

Poirier P, Giles TD, Bray GA, Hong Y, Stern JS, Pi-Sunyer FX, Eckel RH. Obesity and cardiovascular disease: pathophysiology, evaluation, and effect of weight loss an update of the 1997 American Heart Association Scientific statement on obesity and heart disease from the obesity committee of the council on nutrition, physical activity, and metabolism. *Circulation* 2006;113(6):898-918.

Polednak AP. Estimating the number of U.S. incident cancers attributable to obesity and the impact on temporal trends in incidence rates for obesity-related cancers. *Cancer Detect Prev*, 2008. 32(3):190-9.

Polonsky KS, Given BD, Van Cauter E. Twenty-four-hour profiles and pulsatile patterns of insulin secretion in normal and obese subjects. *Journal of clinical investigation.* 1988;31(2):442.

Porte Jr D, Woods SC. Regulation of food intake and body weight by insulin. *Diabetologia.* 1981;20(3):274-80.

Posovszky C, Wabitsch M. Regulation of appetite, satiation, and body weight by enteroendocrine cells. Part 1: characteristics of enteroendocrine cells and their capability of weight regulation. *Hormone Research in Paediatrics.* 2015;83(1):1-10.

Posovszky C, Wabitsch M. Regulation of Appetite, Satiation, and Body Weight by Enteroendocrine Cells. Part 2: Therapeutic Potential of Enteroendocrine Cells in the Treatment of Obesity. *Hormone Research in Paediatrics.* 2015;83(1):11-18.

Prudom C, Liu J, Patrie J, Gaylinn BD, Foster-Schubert KE, Cummings DE, et al. Comparison of competitive radioimmunoassays and two-site sandwich assays for the measurement and interpretation of plasma ghrelin levels. *J Clin Endocrinol Metab.* 2010;95:2351-8.

Rabe K, Lehrke M, Parhofer KG, Broedl UC (2008) Adipokines and insulin resistance. *Mol Med* 14:741–751.

Rabiee A, Magruder JT, Salas-Carrillo R, Carlson O, Egan JM, Askin FB, Elahi D, Andersen DK. Hyperinsulinemic hypoglycemia after Roux-en-Y gastric bypass: unraveling the role of gut hormonal and pancreatic endocrine dysfunction. *Journal of Surgical Research.* 2011;167(2):199-205.

Rajala MW, Qi Y, Patel HR, Takahashi N, Banerjee R, Pajvani UB, et al. Regulation of resistin expression and circulating levels in obesity, diabetes, and fasting. *Diabetes.* 2004; 53:1671–1679.

Rao RS, Kini S. GIP and bariatric surgery. *Obesity surgery.* 2011;21(2):244-52.

Rask-Madsen C, Kahn CR. Tissue-specific insulin signaling, metabolic syndrome, and cardiovascular disease. *Arterioscler Thromb Vasc Biol.* 2012;32(9):2052-9.

Raybould, H.E., Capsaicin-sensitive vagal afferents and CCK in inhibition of gastric motor function induced by intestinal nutrients. *Peptides* 1991;12(6):1279-83.

Rhee NA, Wahlgren CD, Pedersen J, Mortensen B, Langholz E, Wandall EP, Friis SU, Vilmann P, Paulsen SJ, Kristiansen VB, Jelsing J. Effect of Roux-en-Y gastric bypass on the distribution and hormone expression of small-intestinal enteroendocrine cells in obese patients with type 2 diabetes. *Diabetologia.* 2015;58(10):2254-8.

Rocca AS, Brubaker PL. Role of the vagus nerve in mediating proximal nutrient-induced glucagon-like peptide-1 secretion. *Endocrinology* 1999;140:1687–1694.

Rodieux F, Giusti V, D'Alessio DA, Suter M, Tappy L. Effects of gastric bypass and gastric banding on glucose kinetics and gut hormone release. *Obesity (Silver Spring)* 2008;16: 298-305.

Romero F, Nicolau J, Flores L, Casamitjana R, Ibarzabal A, Lacy A, Vidal J. Comparable early changes in gastrointestinal hormones after sleeve gastrectomy and Roux-En-Y gastric bypass surgery for morbidly obese type 2 diabetic subjects. *Surgical endoscopy.* 2012;26(8):2231-9.

Rosmond, R., et al., Mental distress, obesity and body fat distribution in middle-aged men. *Obes Res* 1996;4(3):245-52.

Roth CL, Reinehr T, Schernthaner GH, Kopp HP, Kriwanek S, Schernthaner G. Ghrelin and obestatin levels in severely obese women before and after weight loss after Roux-en-Y gastric bypass surgery. *Obesity surgery.* 2009;19(1):29-35.

Rothenberg ME, Eilertson CD, Klein K, Zhou Y, Lindberg I, McDonald JK, Mackin RB, Noe BD. Processing of mouse proglucagon by recombinant prohormone convertase 1 and immunopurified prohormone convertase 2 in vitro. *J Biol Chem* 1995;270:10136-10146.

Rotondo A, Amato A, Baldassano S, Lentini L, Mulè F. Gastric relaxation induced by glucagon-like peptide-2 in mice fed a high-fat diet or fasted. *Peptides.* 2011;32(8):1587-92.

Rowland NE, Crews EC, Gentry RM. Comparison of Fos induced in rat brain by GLP-1 and amylin. *Regul Pept* 1997;71:171–174.

Rubino F, Gagner M, Gentileschi P, Kini S, Fukuyama S, Feng J, et al. The early effect of the Roux-en-Y gastric bypass on hormones involved in body weight regulation and glucose metabolism. *Ann Surg.* 2004;240:236–242.

Rubino F. Is type 2 diabetes an operable intestinal disease? A provocative yet reasonable hypothesis. *Diabetes Care.* 2008;31(2):S290–6.

Rubino F, Schauer PR, Kaplan LM, Cummings DE. Metabolic surgery to treat type 2 diabetes: clinical outcomes and mechanisms of action. *Annu Rev Med.* 2010;61:393-411.

Russell-Jones D, Gough S. Recent advances in incretin-based therapies. *Clinical endocrinology.* 2012;77(4):489-99.

Safatle-Ribeiro AV, Petersen PA, Pereira Filho DS, Corbett CE, Faintuch J, Ishida R, Sakai P, Cecconello I, Ribeiro Jr U. Epithelial cell turnover is increased in the excluded stomach mucosa after Roux-en-Y gastric bypass for morbid obesity. *Obesity surgery.* 2013;23(10):1616-23.

Sakata I, Yang J, Lee CE, Osborne-Lawrence S, Rovinsky SA, Elmquist JK, et al. Colocalization of ghrelin O-acyltransferase and ghrelin in gastric mucosal cells. *Am J Physiol Endocrinol Metab* 2009;297:E134–41.

Sala PC, Torrinhas RS, Giannella-Neto D, Waitzberg DL. Relationship between gut hormones and glucose homeostasis after bariatric surgery. *Diabetology and metabolic syndrome.* 2014;6(1):1.

Samat A, Malin SK, Huang H, Schauer PR, Kirwan JP, Kashyap SR. Ghrelin suppression is associated with weight loss and insulin action following gastric bypass surgery at 12 months in obese adults with type 2 diabetes. *Diabetes, Obesity and Metabolism.* 2013;15(10):963-6.

Santoro S, Milleo FQ, Malzoni CE, Klajner S, Borges PC, Santo MA, et al. Enterohormonal changes after digestive adaptation: five-year results of a surgical proposal to treat obesity and associated diseases. *Obes Surg.* 2008;18(1):17-26.

Saxena R, Hivert MF, Langenberg C, Tanaka T, Pankow JS, Vollenweider P, Lyssenko V, et al. Genetic variation in GIPR influences the glucose and insulin responses to an oral glucose challenge. *Nat Genet* 2010;42:142–148.

Schjoldager BT, Baldissera FG, Mortensen PE, Holst JJ, Christiansen J. Oxyntomodulin: a potential hormone from the distal gut. Pharmacokinetics and effects on gastric acid and insulin secretion in man. *European journal of clinical investigation.* 1988;18(5):499-503.

Schjoldager B, Mortensen PE, Myhre J, Christiansen J, Holst JJ. Oxyntomodulin from distal gut. *Digestive diseases and sciences.* 1989;34(9):1411-9.

Schmidt WE, Siegel EG, Creutzfeldt W. Glucagon-like peptide-1 but not glucagon-like peptide-2 stimulates insulin release from isolated rat pancreatic islets. *Diabetologia* 1985;28:704–707.

Schorr AB, Ofan R. Simultaneous use of two external subcutaneous pumps delivering insulin and SYMLIN: use of a double-pump system. *J. Diabetes Sci. Technol.* 2012;6:1507-8.

Schrumpf E, Giercksky KE, Nygaard K, Fausa O. Gastrin secretion before and after gastric bypass surgery for morbid obesity. *Scandinavian journal of gastroenterology.* 1981;16(6):721-5.

Schwartz MW, Seeley RJ. Seminars in medicine of the Beth Israel Deaconess Medical Center. Neuroendocrine responses to starvation and weight loss. *N Engl J Med* 1997;336:1802-11.

Shak JR, Roper J, Perez-Perez GI, Tseng CH, Francois F, Gamagaris Z, et al. The effect of laparoscopic gastric banding surgery on plasma levels of appetite-control, insulinotropic, and digestive hormones. *Obes Surg.* 2008; 18:1089–1096.

Ye R, Scherer PE. Adiponectin, driver or passenger on the road to insulin sensitivity? *Molecular metabolism.* 2013;2(3):133-41.

Shiiya T, Nakazato M, Mizuta M, Date Y, Mondal MS, Tanaka M, et al. Plasma ghrelin levels in lean and obese humans and the effect of glucose on ghrelin secretion. *J Clin Endocrinol Metab* 2002;87:240–4.

Silver AJ, Flood JF and Morley JE. Effect of gastrointestinal peptides on ingestion in old and young mice. *Peptides,* 1988;9: 221-225.

Sinclair EM, Drucker DJ: Proglucagon-derived peptides: mechanisms of action and therapeutic potential. *Physiology (Bethesda)* 2005, 20:357–365.

Singhal NS, Lazar MA and Ahima RS. Central resistin induces hepatic insulin resistance via neuropeptide Y. *J Neurosci,* 2007;27: 12924-12932.

Sjöström L, Lindroos AK, Peltonen M, Torgerson J, Bouchard C, Carlsson B, et al. Lifestyle, diabetes, and cardiovascular risk factors 10 years after bariatric surgery. *New England Journal of Medicine.* 2004;351(26):2683-93.

Sjöström L, Narbro K, Sjöström CD, Karason K, Larsson B, Wedel H, et al. Effects of bariatric surgery on mortality in Swedish obese subjects. *New England journal of medicine.* 2007; 357:741–752.

Sloth B, Holst JJ, Flint A, Gregersen NT, Astrup A. Effects of PYY1–36 and PYY3–36 on appetite, energy intake, energy expenditure, glucose and fat metabolism in obese and lean subjects. *American Journal of Physiology-Endocrinology and Metabolism.* 2007;292(4):E1062-8.

Spiller RC, Trotman IF, Higgins BE, Ghatei MA, Grimble GK, Lee YC, Bloom SR, Misiewicz JJ, Silk DB. The ileal brake--inhibition of jejunal motility after ileal fat perfusion in man. *Gut.* 1984;25(4):365-74.

Stenstrom B, Zhao CM, Tommeras K, Arum CJ, Chen D. Is gastrin partially responsible for body weight reduction after gastric bypass? *Eur Surg Res.* 2006; 38:94–101.

Steppan CM, Brown EJ, Wright CM, Bhat S, Banerjee RR, Dai CY, et al. A family of tissue-specific resistin-like molecules. *Proceedings of the national academy of sciences.* 2001;98(2):502-6.

Steppan CM, Bailey ST, Bhat S, Brown EJ, Banerjee RR, Wright CM, Patel HR, Ahima RS, Lazar MA (2001b) The hormone resistin links obesity to diabetes. *Nature* 409:307–312.

Steppan CM and Lazar MA. The current biology of resistin. *J Intern Med* 2004;255: 439-447.

Stoeckli R, Chanda R, Langer I, Keller U. Changes of body weight and plasma ghrelin levels after gastric banding and gastric bypass. *Obes Res* 2004; 12:346–350.

Stylopoulos N, Hoppin AG, Kaplan LM. Roux-en-Y gastric bypass enhances energy expenditure and extends lifespan in diet-induced obese rats. *Obesity (Silver Spring).* 2009;17(10):1839-47.

Sundbom M, Holdstock C, Engstrom BE, Karlsson FA. Early changes in ghrelin following Roux-en-Y gastric bypass: influence of vagal nerve functionality? *Obes Surg* 2007;17:304–10.

Suzuki S, Ramos EJ, Goncalves CG, Chen C, Meguid MM. Changes in GI hormones and their effect on gastric emptying and transit times after Roux-en-Y gastric bypass in rat model. *Surgery* 2005;138:283–290.

Suzuki K, Jayasena CN, Bloom SR. Obesity and appetite control. *Experimental diabetes research.* 2012; doi:10.1155/2012/824305.

Swarbrick MM, Stanhope KL, Austrheim-Smith IT, Van Loan MD, Ali MR, Wolfe BM, Havel PJ. Longitudinal changes in pancreatic and adipocyte hormones following Roux-en-Y gastric bypass surgery. *Diabetologia.* 2008;51(10):1901-11.

Tadross JA, le Roux CW. The mechanisms of weight loss after bariatric surgery. *Int J Obes (Lond).* 2009;33(1):S28–32.

Tang-Christensen M, Larsen PJ, Thulesen J, Romer J, Vrang N. The proglucagon-derived peptide, glucagon-like peptide-2, is a neurotransmitter involved in the regulation of food intake. *Nat Med* 2000; 6: 802–807.

Tatemoto K. Isolation and characterization of peptide YY (PYY), a candidate gut hormone that inhibits pancreatic exocrine secretion. *Proceedings of the national academy of sciences.* 1982;79(8):2514-8.

Terra X, Auguet T, Guiu-Jurado E, Berlanga A, Orellana-Gavaldà JM, Hernández M, Sabench F, Porras JA, Llutart J, Martinez S, Aguilar C. Long-term changes in leptin, chemerin and ghrelin levels following different bariatric surgery procedures: Roux-en-Y gastric bypass and sleeve gastrectomy. *Obesity surgery.* 2013;23(11):1790-8.

Theodorakis MJ, Carlson O, Muller DC, Egan JM. Elevated plasma glucose–dependent insulinotropic polypeptide associates with hyperinsulinemia in impaired glucose tolerance. *Diabetes care* 2004;27:1692–1698.

Thompson RG, Pearson L, Schoenfeld SL, Kolterman OG. Pramlintide, a synthetic analog of human amylin, improves the metabolic profile of patients with type 2 diabetes using insulin. *Diabetes Care.* 1998;21(6):987-93.

Thompson NM, Gill DA, Davies R, Loveridge N, Houston PA, Robinson IC, et al. Ghrelin and des-octanoyl ghrelin promote adipogenesis directly in vivo by a mechanism independent of the type 1a growth hormone secretagogue receptor. *Endocrinology* 2004;145:234–42.

Treacy PJ, Jamieson GG, Dent J, Devitt PG, Heddle R. Duodenal intramural nerves in control of pyloric motility and gastric emptying. *American journal of physiology-gastrointestinal and liver physiology.* 1992;263(1):G1-5.

Tschop M, Weyer C, Tataranni PA, Devanarayan V, Ravussin E, Heiman ML. Circulating ghrelin levels are decreased in human obesity. *Diabetes* 2001;50:707–9.

Ukkola O, Santaniemi M. Adiponectin: a link between excess adiposity and associated comorbidities?. *Journal of molecular medicine.* 2002;80(11):696-702.

Utzschneider K, Carr D, Tong J, Wallace T, Hull R, Zraika S, et al. Resistin is not associated with insulin sensitivity or the metabolic syndrome in humans. *Diabetologia* 2005;48(11):2330–3.

Vendrell J, Broch M, Vilarrasa N, Molina A, Gomez JM, Gutierrez C, et al. Resistin, adiponectin, ghrelin, leptin, and proinflammatory cytokines: relationships in obesity. *Obes Res* 2004;12:962–71.

Vicennati V, Genghini S, De Iasio R, et al. Circulating obestatin levels and the ghrelin/obestatin ratio in obese women. *Eur J Endocrinol.* 2007;157:295–301.

Vilsboll T, Krarup T, Sonne J, et al. Incretin secretion in relation to meal size and body weight in healthy subjects and people with type 1 and type 2 diabetes mellitus. *J Clin Endocrinol Metab* 2003;88:2706–13.

Weinzimer SA, Sherr JL, Cengiz E. Kim G, Ruiz JL, Carria L, Voskanyan G, Roy A, and Tamborlane WV. Effect of pramlintide on prandial glycemic excursions during closed-loop control in adolescents and young adults with type 1 diabetes. *Diabetes care* 2012; 35:1994–9.

Wen J, Phillips SF, Sarr MG, Kost LJ, Holst JJ. PYY and GLP-1 contribute to feedback inhibition from the canine ileum and colon. *American journal of physiology-gastrointestinal and liver physiology.* 1995;269(6):G945-52.

Westermark P, Wernstedt C, Wilander E, and Sletten K. A novel peptide in the calcitonin gene related peptide family as an amyloid fibril protein in the endocrine pancreas. *Biochem Biophys Res Commun* 1986;140:827–831.

Whitson BA, Leslie DB, Kellogg TA, Maddaus MA, Buchwald H, Billington CJ, Ikramuddin S. Entero-endocrine changes after gastric bypass in diabetic and nondiabetic patients: a preliminary study. *Journal of surgical research* 2007a;141(1):31-9.

Whitson BA, Leslie DB, Kellogg TA, Maddaus MA, Buchwald H, Billington CJ, et al. Adipokine response in diabetics and nondiabetics following the Roux-en-Y gastric bypass: a preliminary study. *Journal of surgical research* 2007b; 142:295–300.

Willms BE, Werner JE, Holst JJ, Orskov C, Creutzfeldt WE, Nauck MA. Gastric emptying, glucose responses, and insulin secretion after a liquid test meal: effects of exogenous glucagon-like peptide-1 (GLP-1)-(7-36) amide in type 2 (noninsulin-dependent) diabetic patients. *The journal of clinical endocrinology and metabolism.* 1996;81(1):327-32.

Woelnerhanssen B, Peterli R, Steinert RE, Peters T, Borbely Y, Beglinger C. Effects of postbariatric surgery weight loss on adipokines and metabolic parameters: comparison of laparoscopic Roux-en-Y gastric bypass and laparoscopic sleeve gastrectomyea prospective randomized trial. *Surg Obes Relat Dis* 2011;7(5):561e8.

Won JC, Park CY, Lee WY, Lee ES, Oh SW, Park SW. Association of plasma levels of resistin with subcutaneous fat mass and markers of inflammation but not with metabolic determinants or insulin resistance. *J Korean Med Sci* 2009; 24:695–700.

Wren AM, Small CJ, Ward HL, Murphy KG, Dakin CL, Taheri S, Kennedy AR, Roberts GH, Morgan DG, Ghatei MA, Bloom SR. The novel hypothalamic peptide ghrelin stimulates food intake and growth hormone secretion. *Endocrinology* 2000;141(11):4325-8.

Wu Q, Xiao Z, Cheng Z, Tian H. Changes of blood glucose and gastrointestinal hormones 4 months after Roux-en-Y gastric bypass surgery in Chinese obese type 2 diabetes patients with lower body mass index. *Journal of diabetes investigation.* 2013;4(2):214-21.

Wynne K, Park AJ, Small CJ, Meeran K, Ghatei MA, Frost GS, Bloom SR. Oxyntomodulin increases energy expenditure in addition to decreasing energy intake in overweight and obese humans: a randomised controlled trial. *International journal of obesity.* 2006;30(12):1729-36.

Yamauchi T, Kadowaki T. Adiponectin receptor as a key player in healthy longevity and obesity-related diseases. *Cell metabolism.* 2013;17(2):185-96.

Yang J, Feng X, Zhong S, Wang Y, Liu J. Gastric bypass surgery may improve beta cell apoptosis with ghrelin overexpression in patients with BMI≥ 32.5 kg/m2. *Obesity surgery.* 2014;24(4):561-71.

Ybarra J, Bobbioni-Harsch E, Chassot G, Huber O, Morel P, Assimacopoulos-Jeannet F et al. Persistent correlation of ghrelin plasma levels with body mass index both in stable weight conditions and during gastric-bypass-induced weight loss. *Obes Surg* 2009; 19: 327–331.

Yip S, Plank LD, Murphy R. Gastric bypass and sleeve gastrectomy for type 2 diabetes: a systematic review and meta-analysis of outcomes. *Obesity surgery.* 2013;23(12):1994-2003.

Yousseif A, Emmanuel J, Karra E, Millet Q, Elkalaawy M, Jenkinson AD, et al. Differential effects of laparoscopic sleeve gastrectomy and laparoscopic gastric bypass on appetite, circulating acyl-ghrelin, peptide YY3-36 and active GLP-1 levels in non-diabetic humans. *Obes Surg* 2014;24(2):241e52.

Yura S, Sagawa N, Itoh H, Kakui K, Nuamah MA, Korita D, Takemura M, Fujii S. Resistin is expressed in the human placenta. *The journal of clinical endocrinology and metabolism.* 2003;88(3):1394-7.

Zahorska-Markiewicz B, Olszanecka-Glinianowicz M, Janowska J, et al. Serum concentration of visfatin in obese women. *Metabolism* 2007;56:3095–100.

Zhang Y, Proenca R, MaffeiM, BaroneM, Leopold L, Friedman JM. Positional cloning of the mouse obese gene and its human homologue. *Nature* 1994;372:425–32.

Zhang JV, Ren P-G, Avsian-Kretchmer O, et al. Obestatin, a peptide encoded by the ghrelin gene, opposes ghrelin's effects on food intake. *Science* 2005;310:996–9.

Zhao CM, Furnes MW, Stenström B, Kulseng B, Chen D. Characterization of obestatin-and ghrelin-producing cells in the gastrointestinal tract and pancreas of rats: an immunohistochemical and electron-microscopic study. *Cell and tissue research.* 2008;331(3):575-87.

Zwirska-Korczala K, Konturek SJ, Sodowski M, Wylezol M, Kuka D, Sowa P, et al. Basal and postprandial plasma levels of PYY, ghrelin, cholecystokinin, gastrin and insulin in women with moderate and morbid obesity and metabolic syndrome. *J Physiol Pharmacol* 2007;58(1):13–35.

In: Gastric Bypass Surgery
Editor: Eugene Montgomery

ISBN: 978-1-63485-412-2
© 2016 Nova Science Publishers, Inc.

Chapter 2

BARIATRIC SURGERY ALTERS GUT METABOLISM: ROLE IN OBESITY AND TYPE 2 DIABETES RESOLUTION

Steven K. Malin, PhD
Department of Kinesiology
Division of Endocrinology and Metabolism,
Department of Medicine; University of Virginia,
Charlottesville, VA, US

ABSTRACT

Bariatric surgery has revealed a significant link between gastrointestinal metabolism and obesity that extends to resolution of many metabolic diseases including type 2 diabetes and cardiovascular disease risk. Much of this beneficial metabolic health effect of bariatric surgery can be ascribed to weight loss. However, type 2 diabetes remission occurs within days post-surgery, such that it is likely independent of weight loss. This clinical observation has raised the possibility that altering gastrointestinal anatomy creates rapid metabolic responses that confer normalization of glucose tolerance. The exact mechanism by which bariatric surgery elicits favorable glucose changes remains unclear, but a leading hypothesis is that re-routed nutrient flow to the gut alters entero-endocrine (e.g., GLP-1, PYY, ghrelin, etc.) hormone production, circulating bile acid levels, and gut microbiome metabolites (e.g., LPS, SCFA, etc.) and that favor appetite suppression, metabolic rate, and insulin sensitivity as well as β-cell function. While there is little work in the post-operative period describing the impact of lifestyle modification and/or pharmacology on gut metabolism post-bariatric surgery in men and women, the collective evidence provides strong support for an essential role for the gastrointestinal tract as a modulator of obesity-related disease. Thus, the gut is now considered a novel endocrine organ and a therapeutic target for prevention and medical approaches that favorably prevent and treat obesity related metabolic disorders.

Keywords: incretins, appetite-hormones, gut microbiome, bile acids, insulin resistance and secretion

INTRODUCTION

Lifestyle modification, consisting of exercise and diet, is the primary medical treatment for inducing weight loss and preventing the progression to type 2 diabetes. However, the magnitude and long-term adherence of this weight loss remains low, and with development of hyperglycemia, many people turn to exogenous compounds (e.g., pharmacological/dietary supplement tools) to manage their health. Unfortunately, the durability of these approaches does not typically work well over time in most individuals, and β-cell function declines such that glycemic control worsens. To date, the most effective treatment for obesity that induces substantial and durable weight loss is bariatric surgery. We refer readers to prior work for a summary on the Rouen-Y gastric bypass (RYGB) and sleeve gastrectomy (SG) procedure itself [1, 2], as here we summarize studies relevant to bariatric surgery as a gastrointestinal procedure that promotes favorable changes in insulin sensitivity and β-cell function for glycemic control. Because preservation of pancreatic insulin secretion is a primary determinant of glucose tolerance, we also discuss the mechanisms by which surgery improves β-cell function, and present evidence for the role of gut metabolism in a weight loss-independent way. In particular, we pay attention to surgery-induced changes in insulin secretion that may be influenced by hormones, bile acids and gut microbiota as these represent novel mechanisms potentially governing the rise in pancreatic function.

EFFECT OF BARIATRIC SURGERY ON BLOOD GLUCOSE

Obesity is a strong risk factor for type 2 diabetes. Excess body fat contributes to diabetes development by inducing insulin resistance and inflammation, which in turn, exacerbate β-cell function [3-5]. The notion that bariatric surgery "cures" diabetes has been recognized for over 20 years. In fact, Pories and colleagues [6] demonstrated in 141 patients with type 2 diabetes or impaired glucose tolerance that all but 2 individuals had normalized glucose tolerance within 10 days after RYGB. At 7.6 years after surgery, 83% of the patients with diabetes were off their anti-diabetic drugs, and 99% of those with impaired glucose tolerance were normoglycemic with a normal fasting glucose and HbA1c [7]. In the Swedish Obesity Study, at 2 years post-surgery with an average weight loss of nearly 28 kg, 72% of patients had complete resolution of type 2 diabetes compared with 21% of controls [8]. Many of these patients had been able to stop taking oral hypoglycemic drugs or insulin, which is in contrast to the control group who had an increased need for these agents. These results are similar to those of Scopinaro and colleagues [9, 10] who reported long-term follow up data on 312 patients with type 2 diabetes undergoing biliopancreatic diversion surgery. Their results indicated that 99% of patients achieved normal glucose concentrations by 1 year after surgery. At 10 years after surgery, 98% of the patients were still in complete remission of diabetes (i.e., normal blood glucose without anti-diabetic medication use). However, not all surgical approaches induce comparable glycemic benefit. Diabetes resolution was observed in approximately 98% of patients who underwent biliopancreatic diversion (with or without duodenal switch), 84% who underwent RYGB, 72% who underwent vertical banded gastroplasty surgery and 48% who underwent adjustable gastric banding [11]. In addition, it is also worth considering that more recent guidelines for diabetes remission have been established, and current work suggests that approximately 50-70% of individuals undergoing RYGB or SG may not meet remission criteria at 5 years post-operation [12]. This would suggest that biological factors, such as weight regain or insulin resistance, may contribute diabetes relapse. Indeed, resolution of type 2 diabetes is likely to occur in those with the shortest duration of diabetes (<5 years) or milder forms of diabetes (diet-controlled), lower central obesity, and/or the greatest weight loss after surgery [13]. Conversely, patients that do not resolve diabetes post-surgery are usually older or have a more prolonged surgical disease course [7, 14, 15]. Thus, further work understanding how to optimize diabetes remission rates are needed following surgery. Nevertheless, the majority of these observational studies have been supported by randomized control trials (RCTs) in obese cohorts with type 2 diabetes [16-18]. For instance, the Surgical Treatment and Medications Potentially Eradicate Diabetes Efficiently (STAMPEDE) trial recently demonstrated the effects of bariatric surgery on controlling glycaemia in obese individuals with type 2 diabetes. In the STAMPEDE trial, Schauer and colleagues [19] compared the effects of RYGB and SG vs. intensive medical therapy in 150 obese patients with uncontrolled type 2 diabetes at 1 year post-operation. People were randomly assigned to surgical or medical therapy groups, and the primary end-point was a HbA1c < 6.0%. The results indicated that RYGB and SG each produced significant improvements in HbA1c in 42% and 37% of patients, respectively, meeting glycemic control criteria. Taken together, bariatric surgery appears to result in dramatic glycemic control and weight loss improvements in obese patients with type 2 diabetes.

LINKING GUT METABOLISM TO OBESITY RELATED DISEASE POST-SURGERY

Although weight loss is likely important for gains in insulin sensitivity and β-cell function following bariatric surgery [20], restrictive procedures do not induce comparable diabetes resolution rates as compared to biliopancreatic diversion or RYGB. Moreover, despite malabsorption explaining to some extent reductions in reactive oxygen species and inflammation derived from excess glucose and lipid digestion in obese individuals, nutrient malabsorption does not occur after standard RYGB [21], implying that additional factors likely drive the improvements in glycemic control post bariatric surgery [22]. Altered gut metabolism is currently the leading candidate as the major mechanism following bariatric surgery explaining improved weight regulation and decreased type 2 diabetes and cardiovascular disease risk.

Rubino and colleagues have hypothesized that overstimulation of the gastrointestinal tract by overeating leads to metabolic disturbances that promote blood glucose elevations, whereas restricting food contact with the intestine improves these conditions [20]. A possible mean for improving insulin sensitivity and/or β-cell function is related to the secretion of various hormones released by the gut in response to the re-routing of food intake [23]. Surgical exclusion of the duodenum in the RYGB procedure and exclusion of the duodenum and jejunum in biliopancreatic diversion result in altered sites – or at least altered relative distribution – of carbohydrate and fat absorption. This in turn has been related to increased anorectic hormones that induce satiety (e.g., glucagon-like polypeptide 1 (GLP-1), polypeptide tyrosine-tyrosine (PYY), oxyntomodulin (OXM)) and decreased levels of the orexigneic hormone ghrelin that promote hunger. Based on these observations, the "hindgut," "midgut," and "foregut" hypotheses have been raised. The hindgut hypothesis suggests that diabetes control is due to accelerated delivery of nutrients to the distal intestine, which augments an insulinotropic signal (e.g., GLP-1) that improves glucose homeostasis via enhanced insulin action [24]. Indeed, augmented GLP-1 secretion increases the insulin response to nutrient intake, and at least in animal models, induces β-cell proliferation [25], which together reduces blood glucose levels. In addition to a rapid delivery of nutrients to the distal intestine for GLP-1 secretion, the "midgut" hypothesis suggests that nutrient delivery to the distal intestine increases intestinal gluconeogenesis and activates a heptao-portal sensor that leads to neural signal for reduced food intake and lower hepatic glucose output (26). In contrast, the "foregut hypothesis," suggests that nutrient interactions in the duodenum and proximal jejunum are diabetogenic and, hence, bypassing the duodenum alleviates this intestinal factor that induces insulin resistance and β-cell dysfunction [27, 28]. However, this later hypothesis has been controversial since the diabetic intestinal factor has not been identified and SG, which does not bypass the duodenum, improves glycemic control. It is important to note that although the "hindgut," "midgut," and "foregut" hypotheses are often explained in terms of hormonal changes, they are not exclusive of altered nutrient flow that affects neural signaling. Interestingly, patients following surgery often report a reduction in snack numbers and/or portion size as well as food preference. In fact, these individuals often have reduced preference for sweet and fat tasting foods [29]. In addition, although the gut hypotheses are often presented as mutually exclusive theories, no data actually exist excluding portions of the upper or lower intestine. Moreover, the exact molecular mechanism underlying the improvement in metabolism following RYGB is unknown, and it is likely that as a number of gut hormones and neural signals produced at various sites of the gastrointestinal tract elicit unique mechanisms of action. Indeed, RYGB was reported to enhance intestinal glucose uptake and utilization, leading to overall improvements in systemic glucose control [30].

GUT HORMONES POST-SURGERY: ROLE ON β-CELL FUNCTION

The enteroendocrine cells of gastrointestinal tract are comprised of cells that secrete hormonal factors that modulate not only food intake, but also the upregulation of insulin synthesis and secretion. For instance, L cells are located throughout the small intestine and colon, but are found in highest density within the lower portion of the small intestine. These L-cells are responsible for secreting GLP-1, OXM, and PYY. The release of these hormones, are well characterized, and considered major factors related to β-cell function. Laferrere and colleagues (31) reported increased post-prandial levels of GLP-1 within 4 weeks following RYGB, whereas levels of GLP-1 did not rise with comparable weight loss induced by diet. These findings are consistent with data in patients with type 2 diabetes at 1 year following RYGB in which elevated GLP-1 was significantly associated with insulin action and weight loss [32]. In fact, enhanced β-cell glucose sensitivity (i.e., the relationship between circulating glucose and insulin secretion rates) increase independent of weight loss following RYGB in adults with and without type 2 diabetes [33], although β-cell glucose sensitivity is not observed following gastric band surgery despite comparable weight loss to that of RYGB [34]. Bojsen-Moller and colleagues expanded on this prior work and characterized the longitudinal assessment of insulin secretion and multi-organ sensitivity at 1 week, 3 months and 1 year following RYGB in obese adults with and without type 2 diabetes [35]. Interestingly, at 1 week fasting glucose had significantly declined in patients with type 2 diabetes and this change in glycemia corresponded with improvements in hepatic glucose production since tests of skeletal muscle glucose disposal via the euglycemic clamp, free fatty acid suppression (measure of adipose insulin sensitivity), and pancreatic insulin secretion assessed by intravenous glucose tolerance tests revealed no change. However, at 3 months, while the improvement in the disposition index (i.e., insulin secretion x insulin sensitivity) indicated that insulin sensitivity is a key driver of systemic glucose control, insulin secretion in response to oral glucose was improved in people with type 2 diabetes and directly associated with GLP-1. These latter results highlight that the gastrointestinal tract per se plays a key role in the amelioration of type 2 diabetes. This notion is strengthened by evidence of the GLP-1 receptor inhibitor exendin$_{9-39}$ nearly eliminating the improved β-cell insulin secretion response to bariatric surgery [36]. In line with these observations, more recent work reports that SG produce similar rises in GLP-1 to RYGB surgery at 1 year in both obese non-diabetic and diabetic individuals [33, 37]. These findings are intriguing given that increased exposure of nutrients to the distal part of the intestine is a leading hypothesis for robust increases in GLP-1 post-RYGB surgery. It remains possible that SG accelerates gastric emptying compared to pre-surgery, and this contributes to greater nutrient exposure. Alternatively, other factors in the proximal region of the intestine may play a role. Indeed, it has been reported that both RYGB and SG surgery also increase GLP-1 and insulin secretion compared to intensive medical therapy 2 years post-surgery, although RYGB may provide some additional benefit [38]. However, unlike oral glucose ingestion, use of the intravenous glucose tolerance test suggests that insulin secretion does not change post-bariatric surgery despite improvements in glycemic control [35]. Subsequently, the collective work in the literature suggests that the intestinal system is a key mechanism increasing insulin secretion, and that improvements in post-prandial hyperglycemia occur in conjunction with the disposition index mainly due to rises in insulin sensitivity. Therefore, factors other than GLP-1 alone likely play a role in improved glucose homeostasis after bariatric surgery.

GIP is secreted in the K-cells located mainly in the duodenum and proximal jejunum and released in response to nutrients (mainly lipid). Unlike, GLP-1, GIP is more involved in lipid metabolism (storage) and is thus thought to play a more direct role in the pathogenesis of obesity. While some report similar improvements in GIP between RYGB and SG surgery [39], others have documented GIP levels to be unchanged following surgery [38]. Subsequently, the effect of bariatric surgery on GIP is more controversial than the findings of GLP-1, and the role of GIP is less clear on the regulation of lower fat mass and/or insulin secretion following surgery. Nevertheless, like GLP-1, PYY and OXM are co-secreted by the L-cells of the distal small intestine and are responsible for reducing hunger, decreasing food intake and delaying gastric emptying after meals. Several studies have documented increases in postprandial PYY and GLP-1 after RYGB [40-42], with some also reporting enhanced OXM [43]. Although no published study to date has determined the role of SG on OXM, SG has been reported to elevate PYY and GLP-1 [33, 37, 44]. Ghrelin is a gastric hormone produced primarily in the stomach with secondary secretion emanating from the proximal small intestine, and ghrelin has been documented to play a role in both appetite stimulation as well as impairing insulin sensitivity and reducing glucose-stimulated insulin secretion [45]. Ghrelin suppression is usually improved following RYGB or SG, suggesting that suppression of hunger signals helps sustain weight loss. However, it is worth considering that these surgery types may exert different mechanisms to lower ghrelin. Indeed, prior work by Malin and colleagues suggested that RYGB is effective at suppressing post-prandial ghrelin levels, while SG surgery primarily lowers fasting ghrelin [46]. This phenomenon of ghrelin suppression vs. lower fasting ghrelin may contribute to changes in GLP-1 and β-cell function, although further work is needed. In either case, both surgery types appear effective at reducing ghrelin levels, and this likely contributes to some extent on the beneficial weight regulation and insulin secretion changes post-surgery.

ROLE OF BILE ACIDS ON β-CELL FUNCTION

Bile acids are traditionally known for their role in micelle formation and processing/digestion of dietary fat. However, it is now clear that bile acids contribute to energy metabolism and glucose regulation before and after bariatric surgery. Patti and colleagues demonstrated that total plasma bile acids were significantly elevated compared with weight matched controls in post-RYGB patients [47]. Interestingly, Pournaras and colleagues [48] showed that fasting total serum bile acids are elevated within days following RYGB, but not LAGB, suggesting that bile acids may contribute to weight-independent improvements in glucose homeostasis. Indeed, fasting total bile acids are inversely correlated with post-prandial glucose and positively correlated with peak GLP-1 levels [49] and 2-hour blood glucose levels [47]. In line with these observations, bile acids are known to act on TGR5 receptors located on enteroendocrine cells and promote the secretion of GLP-1 release [50], which may contribute to satiety and β-cell insulin secretion. In fact, farnesoid X receptor (FXR) in pancreatic β-cells may directly respond to the rise in bile acids, thereby increasing insulin release [51]. However, not all studies support the theory that bile acids play an important role in GLP-1 induced pancreatic β-cell function. In fact, recent work showed that bile acids do not rise within the first week post-RYGB and SG despite improved glycemic control [52, 53]. These latter results suggest that while bile acids may contribute to improved gut hormone secretion over longer periods of time, bile acids may not explain the early effects of bariatric surgery on glucose tolerance and GLP-1. Thus, further work is required to understand independent and dependent mechanisms by which bile acids affect β-cell function post-bariatric surgery.

RELATIONSHIP OF GUT MICROBIOTA AND OBESITY RELATED DISEASE RISK

The gut microbiome has emerged as an important regulator of obesity, metabolism and inflammation. In human intestine, approximately 400 bacterial species are present and together resemble a multicellular organ that has evolved to provide complex nutrient signaling and metabolic functions [54]. The vast majority of these microorganisms belong to 3 main groups: *Firmicutes*, *Bacteriodetes*, and *Actinobacteria* (comprising of 95% of total intestinal bacteria) and reside in the distal portions of the intestine. The gut microbiome is a dynamic organ that changes in response to the environment. In animals provided a high-fat diet, the gut microbiota resulted in increased levels of *Firmicutes* prior to the development of obesity [55]. This renders the microbiota to be more obesogenic and may result in increased energy harvest from the diet. In line with this observation, Ley and colleagues demonstrated that food restriction, not macronutrient content per se (low-carbohydrate vs. low-fat), was linked to decreased levels of *Firmicutes* and elevated levels of *Bacteroidetes* [56], suggesting that nutrient overload is important for gut bacteria modifications. For instance, this altered gut microbiome has been associated with intestinal inflammation and systemic insulin resistance [57]. Further evidence for a role of gut microbiome on metabolic health is evident from germ-free rodents, which are protected from developing diet-induced obesity. In fact, germ-free mice have lower adiposity and have higher food consumption when compared with control mice. But when germ-free mice are colonized with cecal content from control mice, weight is rapidly gained and food consumption decreases, suggesting that gut microbiome regulates fat mass and energy store [58]. Further, genetically identical mice fed high-fat diets differed in their metabolic phenotype due to differences in gut microbiota composition [54], indicating that the cause of metabolic disease may be due to a complex interaction of environmental factors as well as gut microbiota profiles. In either event, germ-free mice have reduced expression of CD36 and SGLT-1, which are important for fatty acid and glucose transport in the intestine [59]. Together, these data highlight gut bacteria as important modulators of nutrient absorption, and suggest that two mechanisms are likely involved in explaining the link between obesity and gut microbiome. First, increased capacity to process otherwise indigestible polysaccharides, leading to subsequent rises in nutrients, and second, increased gene expression promoting fat storage in adipose tissue [58]. Thus, a current working hypothesis is that obese animals are better able to extract energy from dietary intake and store those calories as fat. Indeed, obese humans have fewer calories from the diet in feces [60].

EFFECT OF BARIATRIC SURGERY ON GUT MICROBIOTA

Bariatric surgery changes gut microbiota to reflect more of a lean phenotype. Zhang and colleagues [61] showed that microbiota functional differences occurred in obese individuals post-RYGB surgery. In fact, RYGB markedly altered *Gammaproteobacteria* (member of *Enterobacteriacease*), decreased *Firmicutes*, and lowered methanogens (key for energy harvest). Similarly, Furet and colleagues [62] reported that gut micobiota adapted to RYGB surgery by increasing the *Bacteroides/Prevotella* ratio, which was correlated with reduced body fat. Moreover, *Escherichia coli* species also increased in individuals undergoing RYGB, and this change was significantly correlated with fat mass and leptin independent of caloric intake restriction. Changes in adipose tissue mass is strongly linked to systemic inflammation, and consistent with weight loss following RYGB, the rise in *Faecalibacterium prausnitzil* species in people with type 2 diabetes was related to lower inflammation (hs-CRP and IL-6). Together, these findings strengthen the view that obesity and gut microbiota are intimately involved in the regulation of metabolic health. In fact, Kong and colleagues [63] demonstrated that RYGB increased gut microbiota richness, and this change in gut microbiota was directly correlated with genes encoding white adipose tissue mass, metabolism and inflammation. Interestingly, approximately 50% of these relationships were independent of caloric intake, suggesting that RYGB uniquely alters gut metabolism in the favor of weight reduction maintenance. Although distal portions of the small intestine contribute to the majority of nutrient absorption and gut microbiome in humans, the upper portions include gut bacteria that have metabolic function. Indeed, when microbiota from lean individuals are administered into the duodenum of humans with metabolic syndrome, insulin resistance declines independent of weight loss [64], suggesting that exclusion of the duodenum contributes to the regulation of glucose metabolism.

The cause for this altered gut flora milieu is presently an area of intense research, but several proposed mechanisms are currently being investigated. First, the surgical induced restriction in food intake and/or change in food preference, including lower sugary foods and dietary fat, may explain modifications in the gut microbiome composition because of the smaller stomach size and shorter intestinal length [58]. Next, by diverting nutrients away from the proximal intestine, gut microbiota are exposed to more rapid food delivery and adapt accordingly. For instance, intestinal cells are exposed to more oxygen than usual due to the shorter intestinal lengths and facultative anaerobes occurs. Lastly, from an anatomical perspective, pH levels rise after RYGB surgery in the stomach and upper intestine. Although a pH < 4 is potentially "deadly" for many microorganisms, some reports suggest that pH modification affects the overall gut microbiota composition. Further, modification of acid secretion following RYGB not only lowers distal small intestine pH and influences the production of decongjugated primary bile acids, but also increases acidification in the distal small intestine thereby increasing secondary bile acid levels via gut bacteria. Indeed, elevated secondary bile acid levels are reported to decrease hepatic fatty acid uptake, which may contribute to improvements in hepatic triglyceride metabolism and hepatic steatosis [80]. Alterations in gut microbiome in the colon have also been linked to lower pH, and this altered gut bacteria favors the rise in short-chain fatty acid production, which may have lipid metabolism regulatory effects [65]. Taken together, these findings following RYGB surgery support the gut microbiome as being a key physiologic player involved in fostering nutrient sensing for both weight regulation and glucose homeostasis [63].

EFFECT OF GUT DERIVED INFLAMMATORY METABOLITES ON METABOLIC HEALTH

Low-grade inflammation in humans is a common co-morbidity of type 2 diabetes and cardiovascular disease. Locally, the gut microbiome is directly linked to intestinal inflammation via changes in bacterial fragments and/or metabolites known to increase innate immune system responses. Interestingly, these bacterial components and metabolites have implicated the gut microbiome as a key factor in the development of obesity and metabolic disease [66]. The innate immune system has the capacity to sense various bacterial components (e.g., via toll-like receptors (TLRs)) and while several gut derived materials have been documented to play a role in chronic disease, endoxemia by means of lipopolysaccharides (LPS) as well as short chain fatty acids (SFCAs) have received much recent attention as it specifically pertains to inflammatory related mechanisms of glucose regulation.

ROLE OF LIPOPOLYSACCARIDES

LPS originating from Gram-negative bacteria in the gut induces low-grade inflammation and insulin resistance, thereby contributing to disturbances in energy metabolism that promote metabolic disease. LPS is sensed by TLR4, and is elevated in the circulation following high fat diets via a "leaky gut" phenomena (or chylomicron transport mechanism) [67]. This may be of particular relevance for humans, as obesity is associated with elevated circulating LPS levels compared with healthy controls [68]. Human work also supports the LPS linkage to hyperglycemia, as treatment with insulin-sensitizing agents in patients with type 2 diabetes lowered LPS in line with greater rises in insulin action [69]. Further, elevated LPS in type 1 diabetic and kidney vascular disease were highly associated with serum triglycerides, diastolic blood pressure and inflammation markers (e.g., MCP-1) [70], suggesting that metabolic LPS is linked to cardiovascular disease. Given that bariatric surgery alters the gut microbiome composition, it would seem reasonable to suspect changes in LPS. The limited evidence suggests that not only does bariatric surgery reduce LPS, but also this reduction in LPS is directly linked to lower adipose mass and improved HbA1c levels [68]. Taken together, it appears LPS is related to obesity-induced disease risk, but additional work is required to determine if LPS has direct roles on insulin sensitivity and/or pancreatic function.

ROLE OF SHORT CHAIN FATTY ACIDS

SCFAs on the other hand are produced in the colon by gut microbes that ferment non-digestible polysaccharides (e.g., inulin) [71]. The rise in SCFA (i.e., acetate, butyrate, and propionate) levels are important for weight regulation as they are implicated in satiety and decreased food intake, although SCFAs may act as substrate for lipogenesis. As mentioned previously, improved β-cell function following bariatric surgery is in part related to elevated GLP-1 as well as lower ghrelin. The effects of bariatric surgery on gut hormones and gut microbiome would suggest that the changes in SCFA could contribute to the overall regulation of insulin secretion. Interestingly, SCFA have been shown to influence gut peptides, appetite and energy expenditure [67]. Although studies in humans are limited, Arora and colleagues [72] suggested that propionate may reduce appetite. In addition to the effects on gut peptides, butyrate and propionate may increase leptin secretion from adipocytes [73]. This later mechanism may provide an alternative mechanism by which the gut directly communicates with adipose tissue to regulate body weight and feeding behavior. While SCFAs may play important roles in body weight regulation through increases in total energy expenditure [74], SCFAs also act on GPR43 receptors in L cells of the small intestine. Since L cells are also responsible for GLP-1 secretion, it is reasonable that SCFA may influence insulin secretion [75]. Recent work by McNeilis and colleagues [76] supports this hypothesis and identified GPR43 as a modulator of microbiota-pancreatic cross-talk. Interestingly, high fat diet feeding increased the expression of GPR43 and serum levels of acetate. Knockout mice of the GPR43 receptor developed glucose intolerance in part due to inadequate insulin secretion. Treatment of islets with the GPR43 receptor agonist, however, demonstrated that insulin secretion could be restored, thereby providing evidence that activation of GPR43 by SCFA may initiate insulin responses post-feeding. Overall, these data highlight SCFA as an important factor that reduces appetite and/or increases energy metabolism to promote insulin secretion and action following bariatric surgery.

ROLE OF TRIMETHYLAMINE-N-OXIDE

Gut microbiota release choline from dietary phosphatidylcholine where it gets metabolized to trimethylamine (TMA). TMA is transported to the liver via the portal vein and is oxidized to trimethylamine-N-oxide (TMAO). Elevated levels of plasma TMAO, choline, and betaine have dose-dependent associations with the presence of cardiovascular disease independent of conventional risk factors (e.g., blood pressure, triglycerides, etc.) and medication use [77]. Rats fed high choline diets or TMAO diets develop elevated circulating TMAO levels and greater aortic root atherosclerotic plaque without alterations in plasma glucose or blood lipids. Although obesity may influence circulating TMAO levels, dietary manipulation appears important for modulating TMAO, such that high fat and increased meat consumption lead to greater elevated TMAO compared with low fat and vegetarian style meals. Gut microbiota production of TMAO following bariatric surgery is sparse, as some urinary data suggest that TMA is elevated in rodents following bariatric surgery [78]. Increased TMAO levels have also been demonstrated in humans with and without diabetes following bariatric surgery, although lifestyle modification had no effect [79]. While a rise in TMAO post-surgery would be unexpected given the relationship to cardiovascular disease, future prospective work is needed to determine the impact TMAO has on metabolic health. Additional work is also warranted to determine if gut microbiota therapies influence TMAO since this metabolite appears to be independently associated with cardiovascular disease risk [80].

IMPLICATIONS AND CONCLUSION

Bariatric surgery is a proven treatment option for weight loss and glycemic control. However, much of the metabolic benefit derived from surgery occurs within days following the operation. The resulting weight loss from bariatric surgery is persistent in most patients, and this durability in weight loss is considered an underlying mechanism responsible for the majority of glycemic control benefit and cardiovascular disease risk reduction. However, it is clear that gut metabolism has distinct effects on not only appetite, but also on insulin sensitivity, β-cell function, and blood glucose. Specifically, GLP-1, PYY and ghrelin not only impacts satiety but also modulates whole body insulin secretion and sensitivity. In addition to alterations of the stomach, proximal to distal small intestine re-routing of nutrient delivery to the jejunium may contribute to increased bile acids, intestinal remodeling, and changes in the gut microbiome that collectively contribute to improved glucose and insulin metabolism. In fact, identification of novel gut derived metabolites related to inflammation suggests that the gastrointestinal tract "cross-talks" with several tissues (e.g., skeletal muscle, liver, adipose, pancreas) to impact blood glucose regulation. Thus, additional work is required to determine the exact mechanism by which gastrointestinal, neuronal, and endocrine systems contribute to diabetes remission and β-cell function. Taken together, the interaction between the gastrointestinal tract and obesity related metabolic improvements seen following bariatric surgery warrant referral to chronic disease, such as type 2 diabetes, as a "gastrointestinal related disease." Further understanding of mechanisms related to gut metabolism following bariatric surgery, with or without lifestyle modification, will likely promote innovative medical strategies that improve rates of obesity, type 2 diabetes and cardiovascular resolution.

REFERENCES

[1] Rubino F. Bariatric surgery: effects on glucose homeostasis. *Curr Opin Clin Nutr Metab Care* 2006; 9: 497-507.

[2] Steinbrook R. Surgery for severe obesity. *N Engl J Med* 2004; 350: 1075-1079.

[3] Despres JP, Lemieux I and Prud'homme D. Treatment of obesity: need to focus on high risk abdominally obese patients. *BMJ* 2001; 322: 716-720.

[4] DeFronzo RA and Abdul Ghani MA. Preservation of ß-cell function: the key to diabetes prevention. *J Clin Endocrinol Metab* 2011; 96: 2354-2366.

[5] Samuel VT and Shulman GI. Mechanisms for insulin resistance: common threads and missing links. *Cell* 2012; 148: 852-871.

[6] Pories WJ, Caro JF, Flickinger EG, Meelheim HD and Swanson MS. The control of diabetes mellitus (NIDDM) in the morbidly obese with the Greenville Gastric Bypass. *Ann Surg* 1987; 206: 316-323.

[7] Pories WJ, Swanson MS, MacDonald KG, Long SB, Morris PG, Brown BM et al. Who would have thought it? An operation proves to be the most effective therapy for adult-onset diabetes mellitus. *Ann Surg* 1995; 222: 339-50.

[8] Sjostrom L. Lifestyle, Diabetes, and Cardiovascular Risk Factors 10 Years after Bariatric Surgery. *N Engl J Med* 2004; 351: 2683-93.

[9] Scopinaro N, Marinari GM, Camerini GB, Papadia FS and Adami GF. Specific effects of biliopancreatic diversion on the major components of metabolic syndrome: a long-term follow-up study. *Diabetes Care* 2005; 28: 2406-2411.

[10] Scopinaro N, Papadia F, Marinari G, Camerini G and Adami G. Long-term control of type 2 diabetes mellitus and the other major components of the metabolic syndrome after biliopancreatic diversion in patients with BMI < 35 kg/m2. *Obesity Surg* 2007; 17: 185-192.

[11] Buchwald H, Avidor Y, Braunwald E, Jensen M, Pories W, Fahrbach K et al. Bariatric surgery: a systematic review and meta-analysis. *JAMA* 2004; 292: 1724-1737.

[12] Brethauer SA, Aminian A, Romero Talamás H, et al. Can diabetes be surgically cured? Long-term metabolic effects of bariatric surgery in obese patients with type 2 diabetes mellitus. *Ann Surg* 2013; 258: 628-36.

[13] Torquati A, Lutfi R, Abumrad N and Richards W. Is Roux-en-Y gastric bypass surgery the most effective treatment for type 2 diabetes mellitus in morbidly obese patients? *J Gastroint Surg* 2005; 9: 1112-6.

[14] Pories WJ, MacDonald KG, Flickinger EG, Dohm GL, Sinha MK, Barakat HA et al. Is type II diabetes mellitus (NIDDM) a surgical disease? *Ann Surg* 1992; 215: 633-42.

[15] Sugerman H, Wolfe L, Sica D and Clore J. Diabetes and hypertension in severe obesity and effects of gastric bypass-induced weight loss. *Ann Surg* 2003; 237: 751-6.

[16] Dixon J, O'Brien P, Playfair J, et al. Adjustable gastric banding and conventional therapy for type 2 diabetes: a randomized controlled trial. *JAMA* 2008; 299: 316-323.

[17] Mingrone G, Panunzi S, De Gaetano A, Guidone C, Iaconelli A, Leccesi L et al. Bariatric surgery versus conventional medical therapy for type 2 diabetes. *N Engl J Med* 2012; 366: 1577-1585.

[18] Ikramuddin S, Korner J, Lee WJ, et al. Roux-en-Y gastric bypass vs intensive medical management for the control of type 2 diabetes, hypertension, and hyperlipidemia: the Diabetes Surgery Study randomized clinical trial. *JAMA* 2013; 309: 2240-2249.

[19] Schauer PR, Kashyap SR, Wolski K, et al. Bariatric surgery versus intensive medical therapy in obese patients with diabetes. *N Engl J Med* 2012; 366: 1567-1576.

[20] Rubino F, R'bibo SL, del Genio F, Mazumdar M and McGraw T. Metabolic surgery: the role of the gastrointestinal tract in diabetes mellitus. *Nat Rev Endocrinol* 2010; 6: 102-109.

[21] Marceau P, Hould FS, Simard S, et al. Biliopancreatic diversion with duodenal switch. *World J Surg* 1998; 22: 947-954.

[22] Brolin RE, LaMarca LB, Kenler HA and Cody RP. Malabsorptive gastric bypass in patients with superobesity. *J Gastrointest Surg* 2002; 6: 195-203.

[23] Kashyap SR, Gatmaitan P, Brethauer SA and Schauer PR. Bariatric surgery for type 2 diabetes: weighing the impact for obese patients. *Cleve Clin J Med* 2010; 77: 468-476.

[24] Cummings DE. Endocrine mechanisms mediating remission of diabetes after gastric bypass surgery. *Int J Obes* 2009; 33 Suppl 1: S33-S40.

[25] Pournaras DJ and le Roux CW. Obesity, gut hormones, and bariatric surgery. *World J Surg* 2009; 33: 1983-1988.

[26] Mithieux G. A novel function of intestinal gluconeogenesis: central signaling in glucose and energy homeostasis. *Nutrition* 2009; 25: 881-884.

[27] Rubino F. The Early Effect of the Roux-en-Y Gastric Bypass on Hormones Involved in Body Weight Regulation and Glucose Metabolism. *Ann Surg* 2004; 240: 236-242.

[28] Salinari S, Debard C, Bertuzzi A, et al. Jejunal proteins secreted by db/db mice or insulin-resistant humans impair the insulin signaling and determine insulin resistance. *PLoS ONE* 2013; 8: e56258-e56258.

[29] Ionut V and Bergman RN. Mechanisms responsible for excess weight loss after bariatric surgery. *J Diabetes Sci Tech* 2011; 5: 1263-1282.

[30] Saeidi N, Meoli L, Nestoridi E, et al. Reprogramming of intestinal glucose metabolism and glycemic control in rats after gastric bypass. *Science* 2013; 341: 406-410.

[31] Laferrere B, Teixeira J, McGinty J, Tran H, Egger J, Colarusso A et al. Effect of weight loss by gastric bypass surgery versus hypocaloric diet on glucose and incretin levels in patients with type 2 diabetes. *J Clin Endocrinol Metab* 2008; 93: 2479-2485.

[32] Samat A, Malin SK, Huang H, Schauer PR, Kirwan JP and Kashyap SR. Ghrelin suppression is associated with weight loss and insulin action following gastric bypass surgery at 12-months in obese adults with type 2 diabetes. *Diabetes Obes Metab.* 2013; 15: 963-6

[33] Nannipieri M, Mari A, Anselmino M. et al. The role of beta-cell function and insulin sensitivity in the remission of type 2 diabetes after gastric bypass surgery. *J Clin Endocrinol Metab* 2011; 96: E1372-9.

[34] Kashyap SR, Daud S, Kelly KR, et al. Acute effects of gastric bypass versus gastric restrictive surgery on beta-cell function and insulinotropic hormones in severely obese patients with type 2 diabetes. *Int J Obes* 2010; 34: 462-471.

[35] Bojsen Møller KN, Dirksen C, Jørgensen NB, et al. Early enhancements of hepatic and later of peripheral insulin sensitivity combined with increased postprandial insulin secretion contribute to improved glycemic control after Roux-en-Y gastric bypass. *Diabetes* 2014; 63: 1725-37.

[36] Salehi M, Prigeon RL and D'Alessio DA. Gastric bypass surgery enhances glucagon-like peptide 1-stimulated postprandial insulin secretion in humans. *Diabetes* 2011; 60: 2308-14.

[37] Peterli R, Steinert RE, Woelnerhanssen B, et al. Metabolic and hormonal changes after laparoscopic Roux-en-Y gastric bypass and sleeve

gastrectomy: a randomized, prospective trial. *Obesity Surg* 2012; 22: 740-748.

[38] Kashayp SR, Bhatt DL, Wolski K, et al. Metabolic effects of bariatric surgery in patients with moderate obesity and type 2 diabetes: analysis of a randomized control trial comparing surgery with intensive medical treatment. *Diabetes Care.* 2013; 36: 2175-82.

[39] Romero F, Nicolau J, Flores L, et al. Comparable early changes in gastrointestinal hormones after sleeve gastrectomy and Roux-En-Y gastric bypass surgery for morbidly obese type 2 diabetic subjects. *Surg Endosc* 2012; 26: 2231-9.

[40] Korner J, Bessler M, Inabnet W, Taveras C and Holst JJ. Exaggerated glucagon-like peptide-1 and blunted glucose-dependent insulinotropic peptide secretion are associated with Roux-en-Y gastric bypass but not adjustable gastric banding. *Surg Obesity Relat Dis* 2007; 3: 597-601.

[41] Hanusch Enserer U, Ghatei MA, Cauza E, Bloom SR, Prager R and Roden M. Relation of fasting plasma peptide YY to glucose metabolism and cardiovascular risk factors after restrictive bariatric surgery. *Wien Klin Wochenschr* 2007; 119: 291-296.

[42] le Roux CW, Aylwin SJ, Batterham RL, et al. Gut hormone profiles following bariatric surgery favor an anorectic state, facilitate weight loss, and improve metabolic parameters. *Ann Surg* 2006; 243: 108-114.

[43] Laferrere B, Swerdlow N, Bawa B, et al. Rise of oxyntomodulin in response to oral glucose after gastric bypass surgery in patients with type 2 diabetes. *J Clin Endocrinol Metab* 2010; 95: 4072-4076.

[44] Quercia I, Dutia R, Kotler DP, Belsley S, Laferrere B. Gastrointestinal changes after bariatric surgery. *Diabetes Metab* 2014; 40(2):87-94.

[45] Tong J, Prigeon RL, Davis HW, et al. Ghrelin suppresses glucose-stimulated insulin secretion and deteriorates glucose tolerance in healthy humans. *Diabetes* 2010; 59: 2145-2151.

[46] Malin SK, Samat A, Wolski K, et al. Improved acylated ghrelin suppression at 2 years in obese patients with type 2 diabetes: effects of bariatric surgery vs standard medical therapy. *Int J Obes* 2014; 38(3):364-70.

[47] Patti ME, Houten S, Bianco AC, et al. Serum bile acids are higher in humans with prior gastric bypass: potential contribution to improved glucose and lipid metabolism. *Obesity* 2009; 17: 1671-1677.

[48] Pournaras DJ, Glicksman C, Vincent R, et al. The role of bile after Roux-en-Y gastric bypass in promoting weight loss and improving glycaemic control. *Endocrinology* 2012; 153: 3613-3619.

[49]   Katsuma S, Hirasawa A, Tsujimoto G. Bile acids promote glucagon-like peptide-1 secretion through TGR5 in a murine enteroendocrine cell line STC-1. *Biochem Biophys Res Commun* 2005; 329: 386-390.

[50]   Thomas C, Gioiello A, Noriega L, et al. TGR5-mediated bile acid sensing controls glucose homeostasis. *Cell metabolism* 2009; 10: 167-177.

[51]   Dufer M, Horth K, Wagner R, et al. Bile acids acutely stimulate insulin secretion of mouse β-cells via farnesoid X receptor activation and K(ATP) channel inhibition. *Diabetes* 2012; 61: 1479-1489.

[52]   Jørgensen N, Dirksen C, Bojsen Møller K, et al. Improvements in glucose metabolism early after gastric bypass surgery are not explained by increases in total bile acids and fibroblast growth factor 19 concentrations. *J Clin Endocrinol Metab* 2015; 100: E396-406.

[53]   Steinert RE, Peterli R, Keller S, et al. Bile acids and gut peptide secretion after bariatric surgery: a 1-year prospective randomized pilot trial. *Obesity (Silver Spring)* 2013; 21: E660-8.

[54]   Breen DM, Rasmussen BA, Cote DA, Jackson VM, Lam TK. Nutrient-sensing mechanisms in the gut as therapeutic targets for diabetes. *Diabetes* 2013; 62: 3005-3013.

[55]   Hildebrandt MA, Hoffmann C, Sherrill Mix SA, et al. High-fat diet determines the composition of the murine gut microbiome independently of obesity. *Gastroenterology* 2009; 137: 1716-24.e1.

[56]   Ley RE, Turnbaugh PL, Klein S, Gordon JI. Microbial ecology: human gut microbes associated with obesity. *Nature* 2006; 444: 1022-1023.

[57]   Ding S, Chi MM, Scull B, et al. High-fat diet: bacteria interactions promote intestinal inflammation which precedes and correlates with obesity and insulin resistance in mouse. *PLoS ONE* 2010; 5: e12191-e12191.

[58]   Aron-Wisnewsky J, Dore J, Clement K. The importance of the gut microbiota after bariatric surgery. *Nat Rev Gastroenterol Hepatol* 2012; 9: 590-598.

[59]   Swartz TD, Duca FA, de Wouters T, Sakar Y, Covasa, M. Up-regulation of intestinal type 1 taste receptor 3 and sodium glucose luminal transporter-1 expression and increased sucrose intake in mice lacking gut microbiota. *Br J Nutr* 2012; 107: 521-630.

[60]   Schwiertz A, Taras D, Schafer K, Bejer S, Bos NA, Donus C, Hard PD. Microbiota and SCFA in lean and overweight healthy subjects. *Obesity* 2010; 18: 190-195.

[61] Zhang H, DiBaise JK, Zuccolo A, et al. Human gut microbiota in obesity and after gastric bypass. *Proc Natl Acad Sci U S A* 2009; 106: 2365-2370.

[62] Furet JP, Kong LC, Tap J, et al. Differential adaptation of human gut microbiota to bariatric surgery-induced weight loss: links with metabolic and low-grade inflammation markers. *Diabetes* 2010; 59: 3049-3057.

[63] Kong LC, Tap J, Aron-Wisnewsky J, et al. Gut microbiota after gastric bypass in human obesity: increased richness and associations of bacterial genera with adipose tissue genes. *Am J Clin Nutr* 2013; 98: 16-24.

[64] Vrieze A, Van Nood E, Holleman F, et al. Transfer of intestinal microbiota from lean donors increases insulin sensitivity in individuals with metabolic syndrome. *Gastroenterology* 2012; 143: 913-6.e7.

[65] Walker AW, Duncan SH, McWilliam Leitch EC, Child MW, Flint HJ. pH and peptide supply can radically alter bacterial populations and short-chain fatty acid ratios within microbial communities from the human colon. *Appl Environ Microbiol* 2005; 71: 3692-3700.

[66] Laferrere B. Gut feelings about diabetes. *Endocrinol Nutr* 2012; 59: 254-260.

[67] Tilg H, Kaser A. Gut microbiome, obesity, and metabolic dysfunction. *J Clin Invest* 2011; 121: 2126-2132.

[68] Trøseid M, Nestvold TK, Rudi K, Thoresen H, Nielsen EW, Lappegård KT. Plasma lipopolysaccharide is closely associated with glycemic control and abdominal obesity: evidence from bariatric surgery. *Diabetes Care* 2013; 36: 3627-3632.

[69] Creely SJ, McTernan PG, Kusminski CM. Lipopolysaccharide activates an innate immune system response in human adipose tissue in obesity and type 2 diabetes. *Am J Physiol Endocrinol Metabol* 2007; 292: E740-E747.

[70] Lassenius MI, Pietiläinen KH, Kaartinen K, et al. Bacterial endotoxin activity in human serum is associated with dyslipidemia, insulin resistance, obesity, and chronic inflammation. *Diabetes Care* 2011; 34: 1809-1815.

[71] Cani PD, Neyrinck AM, Fava F, et al. Selective increases of bifidobacteria in gut microflora improve high-fat-diet-induced diabetes in mice through a mechanism associated with endotoxaemia. *Diabetologia* 2007; 50: 2374-2383.

[72] Arora T, Sharma R, Frost G. Propionate. Anti-obesity and satiety enhancing factor? *Appetite* 2011; 56: 511-515.

[73] Soliman MM, Ahmed MM, Salah-Eldin AE, Abdel-Aal AA. Butyrate regulates leptin expression through different signaling pathways in adipocytes. *J Vet Sci* 2011; 12: 319-323.

[74] Liou AP, Paziuk M, Luevano JM Jr, Machineni S, Turnbaugh PJ, Kaplan LM. Conserved shifts in the gut microbiota due to gastric bypass reduce host weight and adiposity. *Sci Transl Med* 2013; 5: 178ra41-178ra41.

[75] Bjursell M, Admyre T, Göransson M, Marley AE, Smith DM, Oscarsson J, Bohlooly-Y M Improved glucose control and reduced body fat mass in free fatty acid receptor 2-deficient mice fed a high-fat diet. *Am J Physiol Endocrinol Metab* 2011; 300: E211-E220.

[76] McNelis J, Lee Y, Mayoral R. van der Kant R, Johnson AMF, Wollam J et al. GPR43 Potentiates ß-Cell Function in Obesity. *Diabetes* 2015; 64: 3203-17.

[77] Wang Z, Klipfell E, Bennett BJ, et al. Gut flora metabolism of phosphatidylcholine promotes cardiovascular disease. *Nature* 2011; 472: 57-63.

[78] Seyfried F, Li JV, Miras AD, et al. Urinary phenotyping indicates weight loss-independent metabolic effects of Roux-en-Y gastric bypass in mice. *J Proteome Res* 2013; 12: 1245-1253.

[79] Troseid M, Hov JR, Nestvold TK, et al. Major Increase in Microbiota-Dependent Proatherogenic Metabolite TMAO One Year After Bariatric Surgery. *Metab Syndr Relat Disord* 2016; 14: 197-201.

[80] Tang WH, Wang Z, Levison BS, et al. Intestinal microbial metabolism of phosphatidylcholine and cardiovascular risk. *N Engl J Med* 2013; 368: 1575-1584.

In: Gastric Bypass Surgery
Editor: Eugene Montgomery

ISBN: 978-1-63485-412-2
© 2016 Nova Science Publishers, Inc.

Chapter 3

TREATING THE OBESE PATIENT WITH TYPE 2 DIABETES POST-BARIATRIC SURGERY

Steven K. Malin[1,2,], PhD, Jennifer L. Kirby[2], MD, PhD and Peter T. Hallowell[3], MD*

[1]Department of Kinesiology
[2]Division of Endocrinology and Metabolism,
Department of Medicine
[3]Department of Surgery, University of Virginia,
Charlottesville, VA, US

ABSTRACT

Bariatric surgery is currently the most effective and durable weight loss treatment for morbidly obese individuals with type 2 diabetes (T2D). In fact, up to 85% of individuals experience remission within days to weeks post-surgery, suggesting that the improvement in glycemia is independent of weight loss. Moreover, many individuals see improvements/resolution of their hypertension and hyperlipidemia in the

[*] Correspondence: Steven K. Malin, PhD, Director: Applied Metabolism and Physiology Laboratory, Department of Kinesiology | Curry School of Education, Division of Endocrinology and Metabolism | School of Medicine, 225A Memorial Gymnasium, University of Virginia | Charlottesville, VA, Phone: (434) 243 – 6624 | Fax: (434) 924-1389, Email: skm6n@virginia.edu.

months following surgery. Clinical trials indicate that the resolution of T2D in particular is maintained in approximately 40% of individuals 3-15 years post-surgery and highlights that over half of the people undergoing bariatric surgery may not meet diabetes remission criteria and/or redevelop the disease. Pre-operative clinical factors (e.g., age, fasting C-peptides, medication numbers, etc.) and gluco-regulatory mechanisms (e.g., insulin resistance, β-cell dysfunction) have emerged as clinically meaningful predictors of those who are likely to experience resistance to bariatric-induced diabetes remission. The management of individuals with T2D following surgery requires a personalized approach. Attention to lifestyle (i.e., diet plus exercise) should be the mainstay of therapy while attending to the risks of protein malnutrition and micronutrient and fat-soluble vitamin deficiencies. If these interventions are ineffective, pharmacological treatment in these patients will be an important consideration and should balance the need to control hyperglycemia with the risk of weight gain. A pharmacological approach may also include weight loss agents to combat obesity related insulin resistance and β-cell dysfunction. Collectively, these efforts are recommended to optimize clinical strategies that treat hyperglycemia following bariatric surgery.

Keywords: obesity, insulin resistance, β-cell function, pharmacology, exercise, nutrition

INTRODUCTION

An estimated 347 million adults live with Type 2 diabetes (T2D) worldwide, about half of whom are undiagnosed [1]. Although the etiology of T2D is likely multi-factorial, nearly 80% of all people with T2D are obese, positioning obesity as a key modifiable factor in the development of hyperglycemia. The exact mechanism by which obesity, or excess body fat, induces T2D is an area of intense research. However, inadequate compensation of the β-cells in response to an increasingly insulin resistant skeletal muscle and liver characterize T2D and this is likely the principle cause. Indeed, patients with prediabetes have approximately 20% normal β-cell function remaining and have comparable degrees of insulin resistance to people with T2D [2]. In addition, adipose tissue is considered a chief culprit in the development of multi-organ insulin resistance and β-cell dysfunction through increased circulatory factors (free fatty acids, leptin, etc.) that promote hyperglycemia [3]. Newer understandings of T2D pathophysiology acknowledge that the gastrointestinal tract (e.g., small intestine), kidney, and central nervous system in addition to the aforementioned organs collectively play an important role in the progression to T2D. Thus, identification of end-organ targets that induce hyperglycemia is critical to the advancement of successful treatments strategies, as it seems focus on one tissue alone will not suffice in combating the rise in the diabetes epidemic.

Although controversial, the majority of health organizations consider obesity as a disease [4]. In either case, it is reasonable that current focus be placed on intensifying efforts to improve both weight management and glycemic control to combat the increased incidence of cardiovascular disease (CVD) in people with T2D. Here, we discuss studies relevant to addressing anti-obesity therapeutic options for the T2D individual as well as dual actions to improve glycemic control. To date the most effective treatment for obese people with T2D that induces substantial and durable weight loss as well as improved glycemic control is bariatric surgery. We refer readers to prior work for discussion on the Rouen-Y gastric bypass (RYGB) and sleeve gastrectomy (SG) procedures [5, 6] as here we summarize studies relevant to bariatric surgery as a gastrointestinal procedure that promotes favorable changes in β-cell function and insulin sensitivity for glycemic control. In addition, we present evidence suggesting that lifestyle modification directly and successfully induces meaningful weight loss and increase overall cardiorespiratory fitness, thereby highlighting exercise as a first-line therapy for the post-surgical patient. The present chapter also highlights recent advances in our understanding of pharmacological interventions that may in conjunction with lifestyle medicine drive weight loss and improve insulin sensitivity and β-cell function to maintain/improve diabetes care and obesity management. Lastly, we discuss potential role of these aforementioned treatments in an algorithm for the post-bariatric surgery patient to be considered in the optimization of health care and wellbeing.

TREATING T2D WITH BARIATRIC SURGERY

Several randomized trials confirm that bariatric surgery is an effective treatment that promotes T2D remission [7, 8] and contributes to durable weight loss in part by alternating gut hormones that regulate insulin metabolism (e.g., GLP-1 and ghrelin) [9, 10]. Subsequently, bariatric surgery has highlighted the gastrointestinal system as a key pathophysiologic mediator in the development of T2D. This is of particular clinical relevance given that bariatric surgery (in particular RYGB) improves survival when compared with matched controls [11]. While the literature is inconsistent with the definition of T2D remission, Ribaric and colleagues recently utilized the individual remission criteria of each study to report an overall remission rate of patients with T2D was 63.5% who underwent bariatric surgery compared to a rate of 15.6% with conventional therapy at a mean follow-up time of 17.3 months [12]. The results of this work indicate that people undergoing bariatric surgery are 9.8-15.8 times more likely to reach diabetes remission compared with conventional therapy. As a result of the collective impact of these studies and the literature, both the American Diabetes Association (ADA) and the International Diabetes Federation have identified bariatric surgery as an effective treatment for T2D [13, 14]. Indeed, data support the use of bariatric surgery as not only a weight loss treatment option, but also a "metabolic surgery" that restores glucose homeostasis in people with T2D. However, it is worth recognizing that not all people remain in T2D remission following bariatric surgery and insulin resistance as well as be β-cell dysfunction appear to be key factors explaining the increased glucose levels [15-17]. It is not entirely clear why some people relapse to T2D post-surgery, but some work suggests a direct relationship between T2D relapse and years after surgery [7]. Most recently, a follow-up report to the Swedish Obese Subjects (SOS) study showed T2D remission rates decreased from 72.3% at 2 years to 30.4% at 15 years after surgery [18]. Moreover, long pre-operative T2D duration, insulin use, poor glycemic control despite oral hypoglycemic agents, inflammation, and microvascular complications are all additional indicators of inadequate β-cell function [16, 19]. Moreover, given the importance of sustained weight loss and prevention of weight regain in maintaining durable T2D remission, clinicians must be aware of the various factors that influence weight changes after surgery. Inadequate weight loss and weight regain is associated with non-adherence to lifestyle and dietary recommendations, pre-surgical weight variations, and surgical failure [20, 21]. Additional evidence suggests that surgery type may be associated with T2D re-emergence. Gastric restrictive procedures (e.g., SG) appear to be associated with higher weight regain and lower diabetes resolution rates than RYGB surgery, which may provide a basis for the differential T2D remission and re-emergence rates observed between bypass and restrictive surgeries [18, 22, 23]. Optimal weight loss therefore likely requires greater evaluation of each candidate with regard to their psychological history, as untreated depression, alcohol use, history of sexual abuse and eating disorders have been related to suboptimal weight loss [24, 25]. Indeed, a careful consideration of the benefits and risks of bariatric surgery should occur between clinician and patient prior to surgery such that lifestyle (e.g., exercise, nutrition, support groups, etc.) and/or pharmacology interventions may also be helpful in sustaining glycemic improvements. Thus, while bariatric surgery is a highly effective tool for promoting the reversal of T2D, it does not appear to be a treatment that "cures" T2D in all people. Additional work is required to determine appropriate treatment plans with lifestyle modification or pharmacological therapy for preventing the relapse in T2D and weight regain [26].

POST-SURGERY CARE OF T2D: LIFESTYLE MODIFICATION

A central goal of obesity and diabetes care is to aid individuals in making better lifestyle decisions that lead to healthier body weights. Sedentary behavior and increased caloric intake are two key factors known to trigger insulin resistance and force the β-cell to secrete more insulin thereby over time leading to pancreatic exhaustion and hyperglycemia. In contrast, lifestyle intervention consisting of increased physical activity and low-fat diet inducing approximately 5 kg for 2 years or beyond lowers diabetes risk by 30-60% [27]. Interestingly, weight loss of 2-5% over 1 to 4 years decreases Hb_{A1c} by 0.2 to 0.3%. Moreover, losses of 5-10% at 1 year are associated with reductions in Hb_{A1c} of 0.6-1.0%. The Finnish Diabetes Prevention Study provided advice for subjects to lose >5% weight loss by decreasing total fat under 30% (with <10% coming from saturated fat), increased fiber consumption (i.e., 15g per 1000 kcal) and increased physical activity (30 min/d). This lifestyle prescription lowered the cumulative incidence of diabetes by 58% in people with prediabetes compared with controls [28]. In another landmark trial, the U.S. Diabetes Prevention Program (DPP) Study recommended adults with prediabetes to perform 150 min/wk and lose 7% weight loss. The DPP demonstrated that new diabetes cases were lowered by 58% with lifestyle treatment [29], although subjects who lost the most weight and met physical activity/diet targets had >90% risk reductions of T2D. These reports are consistent with recent work showing that the combination of a well-balanced diet (e.g., low fat and high fiber diet) promoting approximately 5-8% weight loss with increased physical activity is a well-established strategy for managing T2D as higher doses of physical activity generally increase insulin sensitivity [30, 31] and pancreatic function [32]. While caloric restriction is arguably the most important factor driving weight loss, it remains possible that low carbohydrate intake per se may yield greater reductions in circulating blood glucose and body fat, particularly during the first few months during the start of a lifestyle program [33, 34]. Nevertheless, increased physical activity is a primary determinant of maintaining the lost weight. As such, structured exercise interventions in particular have been shown to significantly improve Hb_{A1c} levels [35, 36]. But, whether exercise is effective at improving glycemic control in the post-surgical patient remains unclear, as some evidence suggests that not all people with hyperglycemia respond favorably to standard lifestyle interventions [37, 38] and additional work is needed to define the optimal exercise prescription that sustains lifestyle modification benefits in bariatric patients over time [39].

Although patients undergoing bariatric surgery report being highly motivated for future engagements in physical activities [40], few prospective exercise trials have been conducted following bariatric surgery to provide evidenced based medical practice. In fact, physical capacity and activity following bariatric surgery have been primarily investigated by questionnaire [41-45], pedometer [46], accelerometer [47, 48], or by a short physical performance battery test [44]. In general, the collective evidence suggests that increased physical function to perform daily activities occur with weight loss in bariatric patients [41, 44, 46, 49] as well as disease risk reduction (e.g., hypertension, T2D, etc.) [45]. However, few studies exist objectively measuring cardiorespiratory fitness via whole-body maximal oxygen uptake (VO_2max). Interestingly, in the few studies reporting VO_2max, it was demonstrated that higher fitness levels prior to surgery were associated with decreases in short-term complication and hospitalization stay after surgery [50, 51] as well as increased physical activity post-surgery, which is linked to greater weight loss [20, 21]. Additionally, individuals with reduced physical limitations prior to surgery (defined as an inability to climb two flights of stairs) were associated with greater weight loss after surgery [52]. Thus, it seems clear that pre- and post-operative physical fitness of bariatric patients is clinically important, despite some reporting increased fitness is driven solely by weight loss [53].

Recently, a number of randomized controlled trials have been conducted to investigate the effects of exercise imposed on bariatric surgery to determine whether exercise can effectively promote greater weight loss, fitness, and cardiometabolic health when compared to a standard of care health education group. Shah and colleagues [54] demonstrated that a 12-week exercise program following bariatric surgery improved glucose tolerance. These findings are consistent with work by Coen and colleagues [55] highlighting that moderate intensity aerobic exercise increases insulin sensitivity and glucose effectiveness (i.e., the ability of glucose to facilitate glucose disposal), along with increased VO_2max and mitochondrial adaptation for fat oxidation during bariatric induced weight loss [56]. Indeed, others suggest that supervised endurance exercise or educational based programs with resistance exercise can facilitate greater weight loss, improved muscle strength and increased fitness capacity [54, 55, 57-59]. However, a limitation of the existing body of work is whether these effects of exercise on cardiometabolic health are maintained overtime, and whether exercise is an effective tool for the prevention of weight regain. These are important clinical questions that are likely improve medical practice. Further randomized controlled trials are needed to define the optimal exercise prescriptions that provide additional health benefit as well as to elucidate mechanisms by which these improvements occur.

POST-SURGERY CARE OF T2D: PHARMACOLOGY

Despite randomized clinical trials showing the efficacy of lifestyle modification on weight loss and fitness, long-term adherence to diet and exercise remains difficult. While meeting glycemic goal with lifestyle interventions alone may be challenging for some post-bariatric patients, it is important to acknowledge there are no studies or guidelines to direct therapy in the post-bariatric surgery patient. However, if conventional approaches to improve glycemic control and weight with lifestyle do not work well, then pharmacological agents that target specific pathological defects contributing to insulin resistance, β-cell dysfunction and obesity may be necessary for T2D management in the post-surgical patient. As such, a reasonable pharmacological approach would the one proposed by the ADA/European Association for the Study of Diabetes (EASD) [60].

Insulin Sensitizers

Metformin is the most widely prescribed drug to treat hyperglycemia in people with T2D [61]. In fact, metformin is the first-line oral anti-diabetic medication recommended by the ADA [62]. Current evidence suggests that metformin increases whole-body insulin sensitivity through the suppression of hepatic gluconeogenesis and stimulation of peripheral (mainly skeletal muscle) glucose uptake through activation of adenosine monophosphate-kinase (AMPK) [61]. Although considered weight neutral in most patients, for some patients with T2D and obesity, the use of metformin is of low cost and can promote weight loss [63]. To date, the longest and best study of metformin on body weight comes from the U.S. DPP. Within the first 3 years of this double-blind randomized trial, the metformin group lost approximately 2.9 kg vs. 0.42 kg in the control group [29]. Impressively, this weight loss effect has persisted up to 15 years [64]. Thus, metformin is a logical first-line pharmacotherapy for T2D to manage blood glucose and reduce body weight, although it is worth noting that interactions of metformin with lifestyle are an area of needed research. Studies report that metformin enhances, blunts or has no effect on exercise-induced improvements in insulin sensitivity and glucose homeostasis [61]. Whether there is an optimal combination of metformin with exercise and/or diet remains to be determined.

Of note, metformin is considered contraindicated by the FDA in the setting of renal disease due to a risk of metformin accumulation leading to lactic acidosis. The recommendations indicate that metformin should not be used when serum creatinine is 1.4 mg/dl or higher in women or 1.5 mg/dl or higher in men. In a review, Lipska and colleagues have nicely clarified the many issues raised by these recommendations and have made proposed adjustments to dosing based on estimated glomerular filtration rate, which is likely a better indicator of renal function [65]. Thus, caution should be used in patients at risk for acute kidney injury or significant fluctuations in renal status (e.g., potent diuretic use), based on prior history, comorbidities or drug interactions.

Thiazolidinediones (TZDs)

TZDs act on peroxisome proliferator-activated receptor (PPAR)γ, and are effective at improving both insulin sensitivity (e.g., adipose, liver and muscle) and increasing/restoring pancreatic β-cell function [2]. Despite these gluco-regulatory benefits, many physicians have concern about prescribing TZDs because they promote weight gain of approximately 2-5 kg. However, it is worth acknowledging that this fat storage is in part the mechanism by which TZDs increase insulin sensitivity and β-cell function. In fact, TZDs are known to lower circulating free fatty acid concentrations thereby lowering ectopic lipids (e.g., intramuscular fat) and visceral fat while distributing circulating free fatty acids to subcutaneous fat [66]. In addition, TZDs also have potent anti-atherogenic effects that may lower overall risk for CVD as well as delay the progression from prediabetes to T2D [67]. Thus, given the modest weight gain with this agent, TZDs should be considered as a second-line therapy for individuals who do not achieve glycemic control with metformin plus lifestyle modification.

A concerning side effect of TZDs include the increased risk of fracture, which was found to be increased in women in both the ACCORD trial [68] and in the PROACTIVE trial [69] Given that more recent data has suggested a negative impact of bariatric surgery on bone metabolism [70] it may be prudent to avoid TZDs, particularly those known to be a high fracture risk (i.e., with osteopenia/osteoporosis).

Sulfonylureas (SUs)

SUs increase pancreatic insulin secretion through the binding of receptors related to potassium channels on β-cells [71]. Sulfonylureas are relatively inexpensive and easy to administer making them a popular choice for many patients. Utilization of SUs along with metformin may be prudent for those patients who experience T2D to prevent further β-cell failure. However, it was shown in the UK Prospective Diabetes Study (UKPDS) that SUs had no protective effect on the pancreatic β-cell in newly diagnosed T2D patients over the 15-year study [72]. In fact, blood glucose concentrations showed a continuous rise regardless of SU treatment when compared with control, and this decline in glycemic control was paralleled by a loss in β-cell function (estimated by HOMA-β). This is clinically concerning because by approximately 3 years of treatment, nearly 50% of people required additional pharmacological treatment to maintain Hb_{A1c} less than 7.0% [72]. Given that SU usage carries a risk of inducing hypoglycemia, does not preserve pancreatic function, has conflicting and potentially harmful cardiovascular risk and promotes weight gain compared with usage of oral insulin-sensitizing agents, SUs should be used with caution [71, 73].

Incretin Mimetics

GLP-1 (glucagon-like polypeptide 1) and GIP (glucose-dependent insulinotropic peptide) are incretin hormones that account for approximately 60% of the meal-stimulated insulin secretion, and are important for delaying gastric emptying and reducing post-prandial glucose levels by stimulating pancreatic function [74]. Some, but not all studies, suggest that a GLP-1 partial deficiency occurs in impaired glucose tolerance and in T2D, but there is no resistance to its action. There are two classes of medications- DPP-IV inhibitors that restore low GLP-1 to more normal levels and GLP-1 receptor agonists that directly bind to GLP-1 receptors with agonistic activity that is supra-physiological. As a therapy, GLP-1 targeted therapies have a degree of built-in safety because the insulin secretagogue effect is reduced when eu- or hypoglycemia is present. GLP-1 receptor agonists have two actions that are missing from the DPP-IV inhibitors- substantial appetite suppression with resultant weight loss of moderate degree in most patients and an ability to delay gastric emptying. GLP-1 receptor agonists are more effective in Hb_{A1c} reduction than DPP-4 inhibitors and they are not used in combination.

GLP-1 Receptor Agonists

There are 5 GLP-1 receptor agonists approved for the treatment of T2DM, including exenatide, exenatide extended-release, liraglutide, dulaglutide and albiglutide. Each has been modified to prolong the half-life of the molecule compared to native GLP-1, which has a half-life of minutes [75]. Given the capacity of GLP-1 to promote pancreatic β-cell function and promote significant weight loss, many studies have highlighted the GLP-1 therapy as a novel approach to promote glycemic control and weight loss [76-78]. In addition, a recent meta-analysis suggests that GLP-1 receptor agonists provide more benefit to glycemic control than other anti-diabetic drugs added to existing metformin regimens [79]. Interestingly, studies looking at GLP-1 receptor agonist use with basal insulin suggest that the combination may provide greater glycemic efficacy than either component alone. In addition, the common side effects of nausea (GLP-1 receptor agonist) and weight gain (insulin) may be ameliorated by the combination [80, 81]. Cardiovascular safety trials are ongoing with these agents. Lixisenatide, not currently approved for use in the U.S., was found to be neutral in the ELIXA trial [82], but early reports from the LEADER trial with liraglutide suggest that there may be cardiovascular benefit. It should be noted that GLP-1 receptor agonists have been associated with an increased risk of pancreatitis and pancreatic cancer [83], although this has not been bourn out in the published trials to date.

Dipeptidyl Peptidase-IV (DPP-IV) Inhibitors

DPP-IV is an enzyme that cleaves GLP-1, thereby limiting the gluco-regulatory benefits of this incretin hormones action. Inhibitors of DPP-IV act by increasing GLP-1 concentrations, and are dependent of endogenous GLP-1 secretion [84, 85]. This is physiologically relevant as DPP-IV not only attenuates β-cell function but also decreases insulin sensitivity in adults with metabolic syndrome [86]. While there is limited data on the long-term utility of DPP-IV inhibitors, several studies show that this class of pharmacological agents improve post-prandial glucose metabolism while maintaining insulin levels. Interestingly, this point is consistent with work demonstrating that lifestyle modifications \lowers DPP-IV in relation to lowered CVD risk [86]. Nevertheless, DPP-IV inhibitors have no effect on weight loss, so this treatment regimen appears unique to glycemia per se and may not be appropriate for combating the obesity often associated with T2D during the post-surgery period. Currently, there are four DPP-IV inhibitors approved for use in the U.S. (alogliptin, linagliptin, saxagliptin and sitagliptin). Cardiovascular safety trials in high risk patients have been carried out with alogliptin, saxagliptin and sitagliptin in the EXAMINE, TIMI-SAVOR and TECOS trials, respectively [87-89]. All three agents were found to be safe in patients, but saxagliptin showed a signal for increased risk of hospitalization for heart failure (a secondary end point). The cardiovascular safety trial for currently in progress.

Insulin

Patients with less than adequate responses to oral or non-insulin injectable medications should be considered for treatment with basal and/or prandial insulin as necessary. Although insulin use carries risk of hypoglycemia and weight gain [90], evidence suggests that individualizing insulin titration in conjunction with oral pharmacological agents promotes better glycemic benefit compared to patients who do not respond to other oral agents. For instance, obese patients with insulin-requiring T2D after gastric bypass showed higher rates of complete remission at 1 year post-surgery with personalized insulin titration schedules and metformin compared with patients whose post-surgical medical care did not involve protocol-driven pharmacological treatment [91]. Thus, the few studies that do exist suggest that combinations of existing T2D therapeutics can provide adequate glycemic control during the post-surgical period despite the tendency of insulin use to cause weight gain of 2-9 kg within 6-12 months of treatment [2]. It is important to keep in mind those patients with longer duration of T2D and/or insulin use prior to surgery may have relative insulin deficiency due to reduced pancreatic function. In these patients, initiation of insulin therapy should not be delayed.

Sodium-Glucose Co-Transporter 2 (SGLT2) Inhibitors

The kidney plays an important role in filtering approximately 160 g of glucose each day, and nearly 90% of all glucose is reabsorbed in the body by SGLT2 transporters located in the proximal tubule [2]. Novel data suggest that SGLT2 inhibitors, or gliflozins, are an additional anti-diabetes option that block glucose reabsorption in the renal tubules that in turn promotes loss of glucose in the urine. Canagliflozin, dapaglifozin and empagliflozin are the currently approved SGLT2 inhibitors approved for use in the U.S. for treatment of T2D. A meta-analysis of 25 randomized trials concluded that use of SGLT2 inhibitors for T2D is associated with significant improvements in glycemic control and blood pressure as well as reductions in body weight [92]. This is consistent with other work in patients with poorly controlled T2D showing that SGLT2 treatment as an add-on therapy to metformin improves many of these CVD risk factors [93]. A recent study of the use of empagliflozin in patients with T2D and high cardiovascular risk showed improved cardiovascular outcomes, driven mostly by reduced death due to cardiovascular causes [94]. Not surprisingly, a common side effect of the use of SGLT2 inhibitors includes risk of genital mycotic infections and lower urinary tract infections [95]. In addition, volume depletion and orthostatic hypotension can occur likely due to the osmotic diuresis induced with glucosuria. Finally, the FDA recently updated the labeling of canagliflozin to include a warning about an increase in fracture risk (seen as early as 12 weeks after initiation of the drug) and reduced bone density. The FDA is continuing to evaluate the fracture risk in the other medications in this class. Like TZDs, the use of SGLT2 inhibitors (especially canagliflozin) in the post-bariatric surgery patient should be approached with caution balancing the risks and benefits for each patient. Nevertheless, given the favorable effects of SGLT2 inhibitors on glycemic control, weight loss, and blood pressure, SGLT2 inhibitors constitute an attractive treatment modality to approach management of T2D, especially for obese patients suffering from hypertension.

Weight Loss Agents with Glycemic Benefit

Four new therapies have been approved for weight loss since 2012 and join orlistat for the long-term management of overweight and obesity. These therapies are generally recommended for obese (BMI $\geq$ 30 kg/m^2) individuals or overweight (BMI $\geq$ 27 kg/m^2) people who suffer from at least one weight-related complication, such as hypertension, T2D, or dyslipidemia. With the exception of orlistat, these medications act in the central nervous system to reduce appetite and increase. These agents have been recommended as important adjuncts to lifestyle modification [96] and may benefit those individuals with weight re-gain after bariatric surgery. Many of these therapies have shown benefit in improving glycemic control.

Orlistat

Orlistat is a gastric and pancreatic lipase inhibitor that blocks dietary fat absorption from the gastrointestinal system by approximately 30%. Both randomized trials and meta-analyses have demonstrated that orlistat treatment can produce weight loss and reduce the incidence of T2D in people with impaired glucose tolerance [97]. A recent randomized controlled trial over 1 year reported greater weight loss and improvements in insulin sensitivity in patients treated with orlistat as compared with those treated with placebo [98]. Several mechanisms have been proposed to account for the anti-diabetic effect of orlistat, such as improved insulin sensitivity, incomplete dietary fat digestion, partial stimulation of GLP-1 release, and decreases in visceral adiposity [99] However, orlistat intake is subject to fecal urgency, mild steatorrhea, and flatus with discharge, and the drug may interfere with absorption of fat-soluble vitamins [90]. As such, orlistat should be used with caution to ensure healthy nutrient intake for the patient.

Phentermine-Extended Release (ER) Topiramate

Phentermine is a sympathomimetic that reduces appetite by stimulating norepinephrine action in the hypothalamus. Topiramate is a carbonic anhydrase inhibitor and a monosaccharide that lowers food cravings, decreases lipogenesis, and increases energy expenditure. In the SEQUEL trial, which is an extension of the CONQUER trial, phentermine- combined with ER topiramate induced greater weight loss and HbA$_{1c}$ improvements in patients with T2D with compared to patients treated with placebo alone [100]. In fact, study participants with prediabetes, metabolic syndrome, or both who underwent treatment with phentermine-topiramate had significant weight loss and lowered the progression to T2D [101]. Therefore, because phentermine-ER topiramate appears to induce beneficial effects on weight loss and glycemic control, it warrants consideration as a potential obesity related therapy for T2D.

Lorcaserin

Lorcaserin is a selective agonist of the serotonin 2C receptor. It activates central serotonin 2C receptors with a functional selectivity of approximately 15 and 100 times over that for serotonin receptors 2A and 2B, respectively. It reduces appetite and food intake thereby reducing body weight in men and women [102]. In a randomized trial called BLOOM-DM, 604 patients with T2D were randomly assigned to Lorcaserin (10 mg once daily or twice daily) or placebo, and the majority of patients were treated with metformin, a sulfonylurea, or both. After one year, more patients lost ≥5% of their body weight with Lorcaserin compared with placebo (44.7, 37.5, and 16.1%, respectively). There was also a significant reduction in HbA$_{1c}$ (-1.0, -0.9, and -0.4% points, respectively) and fasting blood glucose (-28.4, -27.4, and -11.9 mg/dL) in the Lorcaserin compared with placebo group [103]. Since Lorcaserin appears to affect both body weight and glycemic control, it appears to be an agent for promoting or maintaining weight loss in individuals. However, future studies are needed to clarify the efficacy of Lorcaserin in maintaining weight loss over time as well as blocking weight gain due to aging or other pharmacological agents (e.g., TZDs, insulin, etc.).

Naltrexone-Bupropion

The combination of naltrexone and bupropion (e.g., Contrave) is designed to target the mesolimbic dopamine reward system and the hypothalamic melanocortin system to reduce food intake. Naltrexone-bupropion induces significant weight loss as well as proportional reductions in fat mass and visceral adiposity [104]. In addition, Hollander and colleagues demonstrated that overweight/obese patients with T2D randomized to naltrexone-bupropion experienced significantly greater weight loss and improvements in HbA$_{1c}$ levels following treatment when compared with placebo [105]. Although these results appear promising for combating both obesity and hyperglycemia in the T2D patient, caution at this time should be considered since attrition rates have been approximately 50% in current trials with the most common side effect reported being constipation, headache, vomiting and dizziness. As a result, further clinical research is warranted to understand the long-term safety and utility of this agent.

POTENTIAL RISKS OF BARIATRIC SURGERY AND CONSIDERATIONS

It is worth acknowledging that serve hypoglycemia has been documented after RYGB and is associated with post-prandial hyperinsulinemia due to elevated GLP-1 levels [106]. This hypoglycemia is classified as neuroglycopenia and seizures have been reported in are rare circumstances. The conventional treatment of hypoglycemia in these patients involves carbohydrate restriction to minimize hypoglycemic related episodes and at times, requires reversal of the surgical procedure [107]. To that end, nutritional deficiencies also may occur in 30-70% of patients. Patients at high risk of developing severe nutritional deficiencies include those who have lost more than 10% of their body weight by 1 month, and those with: anastomotic stenosis, surgical revision requirements, and persistent vomiting [108]. Protein calorie malnutrition is also a concern and can be recognized by signs such as edema, hypoalbumineia, anemia, and hair loss. To minimize these effects, it is generally recommended that patients consume between 60-80 g/d of protein and approximately 800 kcal/d. Vitamin deficiencies can lead to peripheral neuropathy (B$_{12}$), Wernicke encephalopathy (B$_1$), and metabolic bone disease (Vitamin D). Subsequently, in addition to multi-vitamin supplementation, monitoring nutrient and vitamin levels after bariatric surgery is recommended at least every 6 months [108-110].

CLINICAL APPROACHES AND CONCLUSION

The re-emergence of T2D and cardiometabolic disease post-bariatric surgery occurs in approximately 30-70% of individuals. Optimal evidenced based treatment strategies for the obese person with T2D following bariatric surgery is currently lacking, but is likely going to relate to the underlying pathophysiology. In fact, the complicated etiology of T2D highlights that a number of therapeutic options will likely be required in order to correct varying disturbances with tissues (e.g., skeletal muscle, liver, adipose, gut, kidney, etc.) based on the persons age and pre-existing weight status. In this sense, it is prudent to select therapies based on the underlying cause of T2D re-emergence rather than purely on blood glucose concentrations. Moreover, monitoring earlier on in post-surgical process of the disease is likely to preserve β-cell function and restore insulin sensitivity for ultimate reductions in blood glucose and CVD risk over time. In fact, the available evidence and our clinical experience suggest that T2D is related to weight gain combined with the exhaustion of insulin-secreting pancreatic β-cells due to skeletal muscle, liver and adipose insulin resistance. While it is often reported that maintenance of this lower weight following exercise and diet is difficult due to strong compensatory mechanisms that promote feeding to restore energy balance, we propose that exercise and diet is successful at maintaining long-term weight loss and improves glycemic control in hyperglycemic individuals when performed at adequate "doses." Thus, lifestyle modification should remain the first-line therapy for treatment of T2D. However, not all people are able to perform the necessary levels of physical activity needed to maintain metabolic health. As a result, we believe that pharmacologic intervention aimed at reducing weight and increasing insulin sensitivity (such as metformin, TZDs or canagliflozin), followed by treatments that promote insulin secretion if this initial treatment proves unsuccessful, are appropriate treatment strategies. In addition, several of these pharmacological agents (metformin, GLP-1 agonists, SLGT2, etc.) are a viable pharmacological agent for promoting modest weight loss in the obese individuals with T2D. Importantly though, it should be recognized that the quantity of weight loss following these pharmacological treatment plans are modest (1-5 kg) relative to the amount needed for most obese people to achieve healthy weight status and/or optimal glycemic control and CVD risk reduction. Thus, any one pharmacological agent is unlikely to be a sole anti-obesity agent, and these drugs should only be considered as an adjunctive therapy to exercise plus diet. As more patients may redevelop T2D following bariatric procedures, we will need improved understanding of ideal treatment modalities (i.e., metabolic fitness programs via lifestyle and/or pharmacology) to manage these individuals.

REFERENCES

[1]   Maruthur NM. The growing prevalence of type 2 diabetes: increased incidence or improved survival? *Curr Diab Rep* 2013;13(6):786-794.

[2]   Defronzo RA. Banting Lecture. From the triumvirate to the ominous octet: a new paradigm for the treatment of type 2 diabetes mellitus. *Diabetes* 2009;58(4):773-795.

[3]   Malin SK, Kashyap SR, Hammel J, Miyazaki Y, DeFronzo RA, Kirwan JP. Adjusting Glucose-Stimulated Insulin Secretion for Adipose Insulin Resistance: An Index of β-Cell Function in Obese Adults. *Diabetes Care* 2014;37(11):2940-2946.

[4]   Hurt RT, Edakkanambeth Varayil J, Mundi MS, Martindale RG, Ebbert JO. Designation of obesity as a disease: lessons learned from alcohol and tobacco. *Curr Gastroenterol Rep* 2014;16(11):415-014-0415-z.

[5]   Rubino F. Bariatric surgery: effects on glucose homeostasis. *Curr Opin Clin Nutr Metab Care* 2006;9(4):497-507.

[6]   Steinbrook R. Surgery for severe obesity. *N Engl J Med* 2004;350(11):1075-1079.

[7]   Brethauer S, Aminian A, Romero Talamás H, et al. Can diabetes be surgically cured? Long-term metabolic effects of bariatric surgery in obese patients with type 2 diabetes mellitus. *Ann Surg* 2013;258(4):628-36.

[8]   Courcoulas AP, Belle SH, Neiberg RH, et al. Three-Year Outcomes of Bariatric Surgery vs. Lifestyle Intervention for Type 2 Diabetes Mellitus Treatment: A Randomized Clinical Trial. *JAMA Surg* 2015;150(10):931-940.

[9]   Malin SK, Samat A, Wolski K, et al. Improved acylated ghrelin suppression at 2 years in obese patients with type 2 diabetes: effects of bariatric surgery vs. standard medical therapy. *Int J Obes* 2014; 38(3)364-370.

[10] Kashayp SR, Bhatt DL, Wolski K, et al. Metabolic Effects of Bariatric Surgery in Patients with Moderate Obesity and Type 2 Diabetes: Analysis of a Randomized Control Trial Comparing Surgery vs. Intensive Medical Treatment. *Diabetes Care* 2013; 36(8):2175-2182.

[11] Hunter Mehaffey J, Turrentine FE, Miller MS, Schirmer BD, Hallowell PT. Roux-en-Y gastric bypass 10-year follow-up: the found population. *Surg Obes Relat Dis* 2015.

[12] Ribaric G, Buchwald JN, McGlennon TW. Diabetes and weight in comparative studies of bariatric surgery vs conventional medical

therapy: a systematic review and meta-analysis. *Obes Surg* 2014 Mar;24(3):437-455.

[13] Dixon, J B Zimmet, P Alberti, K G Rubino, F. Bariatric surgery: an IDF statement for obese Type 2 diabetes. *Surgery for obesity and related diseases* 2011;7(4):433-447.

[14] Standards of medical care in diabetes-2015: summary of revisions. *Diabetes Care* 2015;38 Suppl:S4.

[15] Khanna V, Malin SK, Bena J, et al. Adults with long-duration type 2 diabetes have blunted glycemic and ß-cell function improvements after bariatric surgery. *Obesity* 2015;23(3):523-6.

[16] Malin SK, Bena J, Abood B, et al. Attenuated improvements in adiponectin and fat loss characterize type 2 diabetes non-remission status after bariatric surgery. *Diabetes Obes Metab* 2014; 16(12):1230-1238.

[17] Wang GF, Yan YX, Xu N, et al. Predictive factors of type 2 diabetes mellitus remission following bariatric surgery: a meta-analysis. *Obes Surg* 2015 Feb;25(2):199-208.

[18] Sjostrom L, Peltonen M, Jacobson P, et al. Association of bariatric surgery with long-term remission of type 2 diabetes and with microvascular and macrovascular complications. *JAMA* 2014;311 (22):2297-2304.

[19] Lee WJ, Hur KY, Lakadawala M, Kasama K, Wong SK, Lee YC. Gastrointestinal metabolic surgery for the treatment of diabetic patients: a multi-institutional international study. *J Gastrointest Surg* 2012 Jan;16(1):45-51; discussion 51-2.

[20] Welch G, Wesolowski C, Piepul B, Kuhn J, Romanelli J, Garb J. Physical activity predicts weight loss following gastric bypass surgery: findings from a support group survey. *Obes Surg* 2008;18(5):517-524.

[21] Evans RK, Bond DS, Wolfe LG, Meador JG, Herrick JE, Kellum JM, et al. Participation in 150 min/wk of moderate or higher intensity physical activity yields greater weight loss after gastric bypass surgery. *Surg Obes Relat Dis* 2007;3(5):526-530.

[22] Heber D, Greenway FL, Kaplan LM, et al. Endocrine and nutritional management of the post-bariatric surgery patient: an Endocrine Society Clinical Practice Guideline. *J Clin Endocrinol Metab* 2010;95(11):4823-4843.

[23] Schauer PR, Bhatt D, Kirwan JP, et al. Bariatric surgery versus intensive medical therapy for diabetes--3-year outcomes. *N Engl J Med* 2014;370(21):2002-13.

[24] Odom J, Zalesin KC, Washington TL, et al. Behavioral predictors of weight regain after bariatric surgery. *Obes Surg* 2010 Mar;20(3):349-356.

[25] Karmali S, Brar B, Shi X, Sharma AM, de Gara C, Birch DW. Weight recidivism post-bariatric surgery: a systematic review. *Obes Surg* 2013 Nov;23(11):1922-1933.

[26] Robinson AH, Adler S, Stevens HB, Darcy AM, Morton JM, Safer DL. What variables are associated with successful weight loss outcomes for bariatric surgery after 1 year? *Surg Obes Relat* Dis 2014;10(4):697-704.

[27] Ebbert JO, Elrashidi MY, Jensen MD. Managing overweight and obesity in adults to reduce cardiovascular disease risk. *Curr Atheroscler Rep* 2014;16(10):445-014-0445-x.

[28] Tuomilehto J, Lindström J, Eriksson JG, et al. Prevention of type 2 diabetes mellitus by changes in lifestyle among subjects with impaired glucose tolerance. *N Engl J Med* 2001;344(18):1343-1350.

[29] Knowler WC, Barrett-Connor E, et al. Reduction in the incidence of type 2 diabetes with lifestyle intervention or metformin. *N Engl J Med* 2002;346(6):393-403.

[30] Malin SK, Niemi N, Solomon TPJ, et al. Exercise Training with Weight Loss and either a High- or Low-Glycemic Index Diet Reduces Metabolic Syndrome Severity in Older Adults. *Ann Nut Metabol* 2012;61(2):135-141.

[31] Houmard JA, Tanner CJ, Slentz CA, Duscha BD, McCartney JS, Kraus WE. Effect of the volume and intensity of exercise training on insulin sensitivity. *J Appl Physiol* 2004;96(1):101.

[32] Malin SK, Solomon TPJ, Blaszczak A, Finnegan S, Filion J, Kirwan JP. Pancreatic beta cell function increases in a linear dose-response manner following exercise training in adults with prediabetes. *Am J Physiol Endocrinol Metab* 2013; 305(10):E1248-1254.

[33] Rock CL, Flatt SW, Pakiz B, et al. Weight loss, glycemic control, and cardiovascular disease risk factors in response to differential diet composition in a weight loss program in type 2 diabetes: a randomized controlled trial. *Diabetes Care* 2014;37(6):1573-1580.

[34] Tay J, Luscombe-Marsh ND, Thompson CH, et al. A very low-carbohydrate, low-saturated fat diet for type 2 diabetes management: a randomized trial. *Diabetes Care* 2014;37(11):2909-2918.

[35] Solomon TPJ, Malin SK, Karstoft K, Kashyap SR, Haus JM, Kirwan JP. Pancreatic β-cell Function Is a Stronger Predictor of Changes in

Glycemic Control After an Aerobic Exercise Intervention Than Insulin Sensitivity. *J Clin Endocrinol Metab* 2013;98(10):4176-4186.

[36] Umpierre D, Ribeiro PA, Kramer CK, et al. Physical activity advice only or structured exercise training and association with HbA1c levels in type 2 diabetes: a systematic review and meta-analysis. *JAMA* 2011;305(17):1790-1799.

[37] Malin SK, Haus JM, Solomon TPJ, Blaszczak A, Kashyap SR, Kirwan JP. Insulin sensitivity and metabolic flexibility following exercise training among different obese insulin resistant phenotypes. *Am J Physiol Endocrinol Metab* 2013; 305(10):E1292-1298.

[38] Solomon TPJ, Malin SK, Karstoft K, Haus JM, Kirwan JP. The Influence of Hyperglycemia on the Therapeutic Effect of Exercise on Glycemic Control in Patients With Type 2 Diabetes Mellitus. *JAMA internal medicine* 2013; 173(19):1834-1836.

[39] Wing RR, Goldstein MG, Acton KJ, Birch LL, Jakicic JM, Sallis JF,Jr, et al. Behavioral science research in diabetes: lifestyle changes related to obesity, eating behavior, and physical activity. *Diabetes Care* 2001;24(1):117-123.

[40] Bond DS, Evans RK, DeMaria EJ, et al. Physical activity stage of readiness predicts moderate-vigorous physical activity participation among morbidly obese gastric bypass surgery candidates. *Surg Obes Relat Dis* 2006;2(2):128-132.

[41] Silver HJ, Torquati A, Jensen GL, Richards WO. Weight, dietary and physical activity behaviors two years after gastric bypass. *Obes Surg* 2006;16(7):859-864.

[42] Bond DS, Evans RK, DeMaria E, et al. Physical activity and quality of life improvements before obesity surgery. *Am J Health Behav* 2006;30(4):422-434.

[43] Bond D, Thomas JG, King W, et al. Exercise improves quality of life in bariatric surgery candidates: results from the Bari-Active trial. *Obesity* 2015;23(3):536-42.

[44] Miller GD, Nicklas BJ, You T, Fernandez A. Physical function improvements after laparoscopic Roux-en-Y gastric bypass surgery. *Surg Obes Relat Dis* 2009;5(5):530-537.

[45] Shada AL, Hallowell PT, Schirmer BD, Smith PW. Aerobic exercise is associated with improved weight loss after laparoscopic adjustable gastric banding. *Obes Surg* 2013;23(5):608-12.

[46] Josbeno DA, Jakicic JM, Hergenroecer A, Eid GM. Physical activity and physical function changes in obese individuals after gastric bypass surgery. *Surg Obes Relat Dis* 2010;6(4):361-366.

[47] Bond DS, Jakicic JM, Unick JL, et al. Pre- to postoperative physical activity changes in bariatric surgery patients: self report vs. objective measures. *Obesity* 2010 Dec;18(12):2395-2397.

[48] Berglind D, Willmer M, Tynelius P, Ghaderi A, Naslund E, Rasmussen F. Accelerometer-Measured Versus Self-Reported Physical Activity Levels and Sedentary Behavior in Women Before and 9 Months After Roux-en-Y Gastric Bypass. *Obes Surg* 2015.

[49] Elkins G, Whitfield P, Marcus J, Symmonds R, Rodriguez J, Cook T. Noncompliance with behavioral recommendations following bariatric surgery. *Obes Surg* 2005;15(4):546-551.

[50] McCullough PA, Gallagher MJ, Dejong AT, Sandberg KR, Trivax JE, Alexander D, et al. Cardiorespiratory fitness and short-term complications after bariatric surgery. *Chest* 2006 Aug;130(2):517-525.

[51] Hennis PJ, Meale PM, Hurst RA, et al. Cardiopulmonary exercise testing predicts postoperative outcome in patients undergoing gastric bypass surgery. *Br J Anaesth* 2012 Oct;109(4):566-571.

[52] Hatoum IJ, Stein HK, Merrifield BF. Kaplan LM. Capacity for physical activity predicts weight loss after Roux-en-Y gastric bypass. *Obesity* 2009;17(1):92-99.

[53] Lund MT, Hansen M, Wimmelmann CL, et al. Increased post-operative cardiopulmonary fitness in gastric bypass patients is explained by weight loss. *Scand J Med Sci Sports* 2015 Dec 4.

[54] Shah M, Snell PG, Rao S, et al. High-volume exercise program in obese bariatric surgery patients: a randomized, controlled trial. *Obesity* 2011;19(9):1826-1834.

[55] Coen P, Tanner C, Helbling N, Dubis G, Hames K, Xie H, et al. Clinical trial demonstrates exercise following bariatric surgery improves insulin sensitivity. *J Clin Invest* 2015;125(1):248-57.

[56] Coen PM, Menshikova EV, Distefano G, et al. Exercise and Weight Loss Improve Muscle Mitochondrial Respiration, Lipid Partitioning, and Insulin Sensitivity After Gastric Bypass Surgery. *Diabetes* 2015;64(11):3737-3750.

[57] Stegen S, Derave W, Calders P, Van Laethem C, Pattyn P. Physical fitness in morbidly obese patients: effect of gastric bypass surgery and exercise training. *Obes Surg* 2011;21(1):61-70.

[58] Rothwell L, Kow L, Toouli J. Effect of a post-operative structured exercise programme on short-term weight loss after obesity surgery using adjustable gastric bands. *Obes Surg* 2015;25(1):126-128.

[59] Huck CJ. Effects of supervised resistance training on fitness and functional strength in patients succeeding bariatric surgery. *J Strength Cond Res* 2015;29(3):589-595.

[60] Inzucchi SE, Bergenstal RM, Buse JB, et al. Management of hyperglycemia in type 2 diabetes, 2015: a patient-centered approach: update to a position statement of the American Diabetes Association and the European Association for the Study of Diabetes. *Diabetes Care* 2015 Jan;38(1):140-149.

[61] Malin SK, Braun B. Impact of Metformin on Exercise-Induced Metabolic Adaptations to Lower Type 2 Diabetes Risk. *Exerc Sport Sci Rev* 2016; 44(1):4-11.

[62] Rhee M, Herrick K, Ziemer D, et al. Many Americans have pre-diabetes and should be considered for metformin therapy. *Diabetes Care* 2010;33(1):49-54.

[63] Malin SK, Kashyap SR. Effects of metformin on weight loss: potential mechanisms. *Curr Opin Endocrinol Diabetes Obes* 2014;21(5):323-9.

[64] Diabetes Prevention Program Research Group. Long-term effects of lifestyle intervention or metformin on diabetes development and microvascular complications over 15-year follow-up: the Diabetes Prevention Program Outcomes Study. *Lancet Diabetes Endocrinol* 2015;3(11):866-875.

[65] Lipska KJ, Bailey CJ, Inzucchi SE. Use of metformin in the setting of mild-to-moderate renal insufficiency. *Diabetes Care* 2011;34(6):1431-1437.

[66] Punthakee Z, Almeras N, Despres JP, et al. Impact of rosiglitazone on body composition, hepatic fat, fatty acids, adipokines and glucose in persons with impaired fasting glucose or impaired glucose tolerance: a sub-study of the DREAM trial. *Diabet Med* 2014;31(9):1086-1092.

[67] DeFronzo RA, Tripathy D, Schwenke DC, et al. Pioglitazone for diabetes prevention in impaired glucose tolerance. *N Engl J Med* 2011;364(12):1104-1115.

[68] Schwartz AV, Chen H, Ambrosius WT, et al. Effects of TZD Use and Discontinuation on Fracture Rates in ACCORD Bone Study. *J Clin Endocrinol Metab* 2015;100(11):4059-4066.

[69] Dormandy J, Bhattacharya M, van Troostenburg de Bruyn AR, PROactive investigators. Safety and tolerability of pioglitazone in high-

risk patients with type 2 diabetes: an overview of data from PROactive. *Drug Saf* 2009;32(3):187-202.

[70] Yu EW. Bone metabolism after bariatric surgery. *J Bone Miner Res* 2014;29(7):1507-1518.

[71] Kahn SE, Cooper ME, Del Prato S. Pathophysiology and treatment of type 2 diabetes: perspectives on the past, present, and future. *Lancet* 2014;383(9922):1068-1083.

[72] Matthews DR, Cull CA, Stratton IM, Holman RR, Turner RC. UKPDS 26: Sulphonylurea failure in non-insulin-dependent diabetic patients over six years. UK Prospective Diabetes Study (UKPDS) Group. *Diabet Med* 1998;15(4):297-303.

[73] Bennett WL, Maruthur NM, Singh S, et al. Comparative effectiveness and safety of medications for type 2 diabetes: an update including new drugs and 2-drug combinations. *Ann Intern Med* 2011;154(9):602-613.

[74] Holst J, Vilsbll T, Deacon C. The incretin system and its role in type 2 diabetes mellitus. *Mol Cell Endocrinol* 2009;297(1-2):127-136.

[75] Gil-Lozano M, Mingomataj EL, Wu WK, Ridout SA, Brubaker PL. Circadian secretion of the intestinal hormone GLP-1 by the rodent L cell. *Diabetes* 2014;63(11):3674-3685.

[76] Pi Sunyer X, Blackburn G, Brancati F, et al. Reduction in weight and cardiovascular disease risk factors in individuals with type 2 diabetes: one-year results of the look AHEAD trial. *Diabetes Care* 2007;30(6):1374-1383.

[77] Davies MJ, Bergenstal R, Bode B, Kushner RF, Lewin A, Skjoth TV, et al. Efficacy of Liraglutide for Weight Loss Among Patients With Type 2 Diabetes: The SCALE Diabetes Randomized Clinical Trial. *JAMA* 2015;314(7):687-699.

[78] Wadden TA, Hollander P, Klein S, et al. Weight maintenance and additional weight loss with liraglutide after low-calorie-diet-induced weight loss: the SCALE Maintenance randomized study. *Int J Obes (Lond)* 2013;37(11):1443-1451.

[79] Liu SC, Tu YK, Chien MN. Chien KL. Effect of antidiabetic agents added to metformin on glycaemic control, hypoglycaemia and weight change in patients with type 2 diabetes: a network meta-analysis. *Diabetes Obes Metab* 2012;14(9):810-820.

[80] Buse JB, Bergenstal RM, Glass LC, et al. Use of twice-daily exenatide in Basal insulin-treated patients with type 2 diabetes: a randomized, controlled trial. *Ann Intern Med* 201118;154(2):103-112.

[81] Gough SC, Bode B, Woo V, et al. Efficacy and safety of a fixed-ratio combination of insulin degludec and liraglutide (IDegLira) compared with its components given alone: results of a phase 3, open-label, randomised, 26-week, treat-to-target trial in insulin-naive patients with type 2 diabetes. *Lancet Diabetes Endocrinol* 2014;2(11):885-893.

[82] Pfeffer MA, Claggett B, Diaz R, et al. Lixisenatide in Patients with Type 2 Diabetes and Acute Coronary Syndrome. *N Engl J Med* 2015;373(23):2247-2257.

[83] Ryder RE. The potential risks of pancreatitis and pancreatic cancer with GLP-1-based therapies are far outweighed by the proven and potential (cardiovascular) benefits. *Diabet Med* 2013;30(10):1148-1155.

[84] Shah Z, Kampfrath T, Deiuliis J, et al. Long-term dipeptidyl-peptidase 4 inhibition reduces atherosclerosis and inflammation via effects on monocyte recruitment and chemotaxis. *Circulation* 2011;124(21):2338-2349.

[85] Shah P, Ardestani A, Dharmadhikari G, et al. The DPP-4 inhibitor linagliptin restores beta-cell function and survival in human isolated islets through GLP-1 stabilization. *J Clin Endocrinol Metab* 2013;98(7):E1163-72.

[86] Malin SK, Huang H, Mulya A, Kashyap SR, Kirwan JP. Lower dipeptidyl peptidase-4 following exercise training plus weight loss is related to increased insulin sensitivity in adults with metabolic syndrome. *Peptides* 2013;47:142-147.

[87] White WB, Cannon CP, Heller SR, Nissen SE, Bergenstal RM, Bakris GL, et al. Alogliptin after acute coronary syndrome in patients with type 2 diabetes. *N Engl J Med* 2013;369(14):1327-1335.

[88] Scirica BM, Bhatt DL, Braunwald E, et al. Saxagliptin and cardiovascular outcomes in patients with type 2 diabetes mellitus. *N Engl J Med* 2013;369(14):1317-1326.

[89] Green JB, Bethel MA, Armstrong PW, et al. Effect of Sitagliptin on Cardiovascular Outcomes in Type 2 Diabetes. *N Engl J Med* 2015;373(3):232-242.

[90] Yanovski SZ, Yanovski JA. Long-term drug treatment for obesity: a systematic and clinical review. *JAMA* 2014;311(1):74-86.

[91] Fenske WK, Pournaras DJ, Aasheim ET, Miras AD, Scopinaro N, Scholtz S, et al. Can a protocol for glycaemic control improve type 2 diabetes outcomes after gastric bypass? *Obes Surg* 2012;22(1):90-96.

[92]   Monami M, Nardini C, Mannucci E. Efficacy and safety of sodium glucose co-transport-2 inhibitors in type 2 diabetes: a meta-analysis of randomized clinical trials. *Diabetes Obes Metab* 2014;16(5):457-466.

[93]   Bailey CJ, Gross JL, Pieters A, Bastien A, List JF. Effect of dapagliflozin in patients with type 2 diabetes who have inadequate glycaemic control with metformin: a randomised, double-blind, placebo-controlled trial. *Lancet* 2010;375(9733):2223-2233.

[94]   Zinman B, Wanner C, Lachin JM, et al. Empagliflozin, Cardiovascular Outcomes, and Mortality in Type 2 Diabetes. *N Engl J Med* 2015;373(22):2117-2128.

[95]   Vasilakou D, Karagiannis T, Athanasiadou E, et al. Sodium-glucose cotransporter 2 inhibitors for type 2 diabetes: a systematic review and meta-analysis. *Ann Intern Med* 2013;159(4):262-274.

[96]   Apovian CM, Aronne LJ, Bessesen DH, et al. Pharmacological management of obesity: an endocrine Society clinical practice guideline. *J Clin Endocrinol Metab* 2015;100(2):342-362.

[97]   Torgerson JS, Hauptman J, Boldrin MN, Sjostrom L. XENical in the prevention of diabetes in obese subjects (XENDOS) study: a randomized study of orlistat as an adjunct to lifestyle changes for the prevention of type 2 diabetes in obese patients. *Diabetes Care* 2004;27(1):155-161.

[98]   Derosa G, Cicero AF, D'Angelo A, Fogari E, Maffioli P. Effects of 1-year orlistat treatment compared to placebo on insulin resistance parameters in patients with type 2 diabetes. *J Clin Pharm Ther* 2012;37(2):187-195.

[99]   Scheen AJ, Van Gaal LF. Combating the dual burden: therapeutic targeting of common pathways in obesity and type 2 diabetes. *Lancet Diabetes Endocrinol* 2014;2(11):911-922.

[100] Garvey WT, Ryan DH, Look M, et al. Two-year sustained weight loss and metabolic benefits with controlled-release phentermine/topiramate in obese and overweight adults (SEQUEL): a randomized, placebo-controlled, phase 3 extension study. *Am J Clin Nutr* 2012;95(2):297-308.

[101] Garvey WT, Ryan DH, Henry R, et al. Prevention of type 2 diabetes in subjects with prediabetes and metabolic syndrome treated with phentermine and topiramate extended release. *Diabetes Care* 2014;37(4):912-921.

[102] Martin CK, Redman LM, Zhang J, et al. Lorcaserin, a 5-HT(2C) receptor agonist, reduces body weight by decreasing energy intake without influencing energy expenditure. *J Clin Endocrinol Metab* 2011;96(3):837-845.

[103] O'Neil PM, Smith SR, Weissman NJ, et al. Randomized placebo-controlled clinical trial of lorcaserin for weight loss in type 2 diabetes mellitus: the BLOOM-DM study. *Obesity* 2012;20(7):1426-1436.

[104] Smith SR, Fujioka K, Gupta AK, et al. Combination therapy with naltrexone and bupropion for obesity reduces total and visceral adiposity. *Diabetes Obes Metab* 2013;15(9):863-866.

[105] Hollander P, Gupta AK, Plodkowski R, et al. Effects of naltrexone sustained-release/bupropion sustained-release combination therapy on body weight and glycemic parameters in overweight and obese patients with type 2 diabetes. *Diabetes Care* 2013;36(12):4022-4029.

[106] Service G, Thompson G, Service FJ, Andrews J, Collazo Clavell M, Lloyd R. Hyperinsulinemic hypoglycemia with nesidioblastosis after gastric-bypass surgery. *N Engl J Med* 2005;353(3):249-254.

[107] Goldfine AB, Mun EC, Devine E, et al. Patients with neuroglycopenia after gastric bypass surgery have exaggerated incretin and insulin secretory responses to a mixed meal. *J Clin Endocrinol Metab* 2007;92(12):4678-4685.

[108] Davies DJ, Baxter JM. Nutritional deficiencies after bariatric surgery. *Obesity Surg* 2007;17(9):1150-1158.

[109] Ritz P, Becouarn G, Douay O, Salle A, Topart P, Rohmer V. Gastric bypass is not associated with protein malnutrition in morbidly obese patients. *Obesity Surg* 2009;19(7):840-844.

[110] Angstadt J, Bodziner R. Peripheral polyneuropathy from thiamine deficiency following laparoscopic Roux-en-Y gastric bypass. *Obesity Surg* 2005;15(6):890-892.

In: Gastric Bypass Surgery
Editor: Eugene Montgomery

ISBN: 978-1-63485-412-2
© 2016 Nova Science Publishers, Inc.

Chapter 4

GASTRIC BYPASS SURGERY AND THE SKIN

Katherine Fiala, MD and Ryan Batson, BS
Scott and White Hospital, Texas A&M Health Science Center
College of Medicine, Temple, TX, US

ABSTRACT

Gastric bypass surgery can affect the skin in both positive and negative ways. Recently, the positive outcomes have been demonstrated with psoriasis, necrobiosis lipoidica, acanthosis nigricans, and hidradenitis suppurativa. In this chapter, we will discuss the recent findings of the relationship between gastric bypass and these four skin disorders. On the other hand, with aims to achieve radical weight reduction, bariatric surgery can be accompanied by nutrient insufficiencies and metabolic imbalances that affect the skin. Such deficiencies can lead to changes in the skin's micro-architecture which can, in turn, affect processes such as wound healing. Changes in the skin's immunity and defense mechanisms can result from vitamin and nutrient deficiency. The nutrient deficiencies are thought to be a result of a combination of decreased food intake, changes in the digestive system's anatomy, and high levels of oxidative stress that interfere with the absorptive process. This chapter will explore the most prominent metabolic and nutritional deficiencies that have dermatologic manifestations including: iron, biotin, zinc, copper, and vitamins B3, A, C, and K. Interestingly, patients may be compliant with their oral nutritional supplements, but the absorption is decreased resulting in low circulating levels. This can, moreover, result in skin and systemic manifestations. Recognizing various skin changes secondary to nutrient deficiency in post bariatric surgery patients is a valuable asset in providing comprehensive care.

BENEFITS TO THE SKIN

Psoriasis

Psoriasis is a common chronic inflammatory condition characterized by high epithelial cell turnover. The classic cutaneous manifestation includes red patches with overlying thick, silvery scales, which may be itchy. The distribution is often symmetrical and shows predilection for the elbows, knees, scalp, and nails (Farias, 2012). Obesity is noted to be a major risk factor for psoriasis. Perhaps one of the greatest contributions to the increased incidence of psoriasis in the obese patient population is the chronic inflammatory state imposed on the body. Psoriasis is regarded as a systemic autoimmune disease in which leukocytes, inflammatory cytokines, and dendritic cells play a role (Faurschou 2011). Pro-inflammatory cytokines such as tumor necrosis factor (TNF) alpha, interleukin (IL)-1, IL-6, IL-8 and leptin synthesized by adipose tissue are over expressed in obesity (Hector, 2014). Furthermore, the severity of psoriasis is associated with the degree of obesity observed. Hossler et al. noted that almost two-thirds of their 24 patients with psoriasis self-reported postoperative improvement after undergoing weight loss surgery. In addition, this study demonstrated an improved response to psoriasis treatment after surgery (Hossler 2013).

Interestingly, while it is no surprise that drastic weight loss after the surgery reduces symptoms of psoriasis, marked clinical improvement may be noted immediately following the procedure even before significant weight loss is achieved. The suspected mechanism involves the glucose lowering gut incretin hormone, glucagon-like peptide-1 (GLP-1). After gastric bypass, the levels of postprandial GLP-1 may increase up to 20 fold (Faurschou 2011). This hormone is not, however, increased in the purely restrictive surgeries, including gastric band or sleeve. GLP-1 is found in the epithelium of the intestinal tract with the greatest density located in the ileum. It is secreted in response to the presence of nutrients in the intestinal lumen (Holst 2007). The GLP-1 receptors on pancreatic beta cells have been shown to enhance all steps of insulin biosynthesis and insulin gene transcription as well as beta cell mass (in cell and animal studies). GLP-1 also inhibits the secretion of glucagon from alpha cells. It is the cumulative effects on insulin and glucagon that ultimately inhibit hepatic glucose production (Faurschou 2011). Lastly, GLP-1 reduces appetite, gastrointestinal motility, and empting. These effects ultimately lead to decreased food intake.

In addition to contributing to glucose homeostasis, gut motility, and satiety, GLP-1 has been shown to have some anti-inflammatory effects. It is this implication as an immunological modulator that provides an additional contribution to the improvement of psoriasis postoperatively (Faurshcou 2011). Its anti-inflammatory actions include decreased expression of cytokines induced by TNF-alpha. This is of special interest when understanding the mechanism of psoriasis resolution. TNF-alpha promotes inflammation through the pro-survival transcription factor NF-kB (Pasparakis 2009). Although data on immunological effects of GLP-1 are still primarily based on *in vitro* and animal models, new and exciting data are emerging. The potential immunological effects pose a link between bariatric surgery, GLP-1 and psoriasis.

Ultimately, it is the additive effects of improved glucose homeostasis, increased weight loss, and reduced inflammation that result in improved psoriasis. Farias et al. reported that seven of the 10 patients in their study remained in remission six months after surgery. Seventy-five percent of these patients were previously taking systemic medications including: acitretin, methotrexate, and cyclosporine. By achieving resolution of psoriasis with a bariatric procedure, serious side effects of these systemic medications may be avoided (Farias 2012). Despite the fact that psoriasis is not considered a life-threatening illness, it is associated with stigmatizing chronic lesions that affect a patient's physical and psychological morbidity. Gastric bypass, therefore, may provide an effective means of treating patients with refractory psoriasis and, ultimately, significantly contribute to an improved quality of life.

Necrobiosis Lipoidica

Necrobiosis lipoidica (NL), a granulcmatous skin disease, is commonly associated with diabetes mellitus. It is typically observed bilaterally on patients' shins, but may also be seen on the forearms, hands and trunk. In the initial stages, the lesions are typically asymptomatic but may become tender and ulcerate over time or when injured. The initial presenting symptom is the appearance of an "erythematous ecchymosis." The lesions are red-brown and indurated with smooth, atrophic central portions. Over time, the chronic disease may lead to ulceration which can then cause dysethesia, pain, secondary infection and cosmetically sensitive scarring (Weismann 2004).

While the etiology of NL is still largely unknown, some of the proposed mechanisms implicated include: T cell involvement, microangiopathy, and immune complex vasculitis resulting in a release of pro-inflammatory cytokines and abnormal collagen production (Sehgal 2011).

The diagnosis is made by punch biopsy demonstrating superficial and deep perivascular and interstitial mixed inflammatory cell infiltrates including: lymphocytes, plasma cells, multinucleated histiocytes, and eosinophils in the dermis and subcutis. Necrotic areas with collagen degeneration in the deep dermis, peripheral fibrosis, and subcutaneous tissue panniculitis may also be diagnostic (Patsatsi 2011).

A very poor response to treatments, including topical and systemic steroids, nicotinamide, pentoxifylline, tretinoin, TNF alpha inhibitors, mycophenolate mofetil, thalidomide, cyclosporine, tacrolimus, and antimalarials, is typically observed in most patients with this condition (Bozkurt 2013; Patsatsi, 2011). Case reports, however, have detected symptomatic, morphologic, and histopathologic remission of NL after bariatric surgery (Bozkurt 2013). It is believed that the significant improvement of a patient's NL is secondary to type 2 diabetes mellitus remission (Bozkurt 2013). This provides a promising therapeutic option for morbidly obese patients with NL who failed medical therapy.

Acanthosis Nigricans

Acanthosis nigricans is a common dermatologic manifestation of obesity, insulin resistance, and consequent hyperinsulinemia. It is classically a symmetrical hyperpigmented, velvety plaque that may occur in almost any location. The most common regions affected include the posterior neck, axilla, and groin. Additionally, less common regions include the knuckles, elbows, and face (Atwa 2014). The skin has abundant insulin-like growth factor-1 (IGF-1) receptors on the keratinocyte surface membrane. Acanthosis nigricans is a common feature in severe insulin resistance, in patients with insulin receptor disorders, and hyperinsulinemia (Babieri 1983; Pugeat 2000; Cruz 1992; Stuart 1986). Large amounts of unbound insulin are free to bind IGF-1 receptors on keratinocytes or fibroblasts, leading to proliferation of the epidermis (Barbieri 1983). Reduced fasting insulin and C-peptide levels suggest that daily insulin levels status post gastric bypass surgery are likely secondary to reduced free fatty acids, leptin, or gut incretins. Moreover, the dramatic decrease of circulating leptin occurring after gastric bypass may contribute to reduced acanthosis nigricans and hyperandrogenism. Androgens target the skin and lead to hair growth and sebum secretion. Increased secretion of testosterone, the main active androgen, can lead to dermatologic manifestations including hirsutism, acne, alopecia, and acanthosis nigricans. A decrease in androgens by the aforementioned mechanism, in addition to decreased active androgen synthesis in human adipose tissue, leads to improvement of acanthosis nigricans. In summary, the combined effects of decreased insulin resistance in addition to reduced levels of systemic androgens results in the improvement of acanthosis nigricans.

Hidradenitis Suppurativa

Hidradenitis suppurativa (HS) and acne inversa are chronic relapsing, scarring skin conditions involving the follicular and pilosebaceous units, which have a damaging impact on patients' quality of life. Diagnostic criteria for HS is clinical and must meet the following three criteria: typical lesions (deep-seated painful nodules, abscesses, draining sinuses, bridged scars, and open comedones within secondary lesions); typical topography in one or more of the predilected areas (intertrigionus skin of the axillary, inguinal, genital, perineal, or infra-mammary regions); and chronicity and recurrence (Revuz 2016; Margesson 2014). The myriad of complications that may result include anal and perianal fistulae, arthropathy, lymphedema, and, even, squamous cell carcinoma of the buttocks and perineum.

Lack of early detection, accurate diagnosis, and proper therapy resulting in relapsing and severe HS is a common occurrence. The influence of endogenous reproductive hormones, exogenous hormones and androgens lead to keratin plugging and distention of the follicular unit. Shearing forces, friction, and pressure ultimately lead to rupture and leakage of the ductal contents, resulting in an inflammatory reaction that is mediated by the innate immune system (Margesson 2014). Given this pathophysiology, the chronic state of inflammation observed in obesity makes it an obvious risk factor for this condition. Additionally, in obesity, the hyperandrogenism, elevated insulin, and elevated IGF-1 activate androgen receptors that control growth. As a result, there is uncontrolled cellular proliferation and subsequent follicular duct plugging. The role of obesity in the pathophysiology of HS was further supported by Thomas et al. in a case report of a man who experienced rapid improvement of long-standing, treatment-resistant HS after bariatric surgical intervention (gastric sleeve) and subsequent drastic weight loss. The improvement was noted within weeks of the surgical intervention, and the patient remained in remission for over a year following the procedure (Thomas 2014). This highlights the rationale that weight loss plays an important role in the intervention of HS and, ultimately, the prevention of the more severe complications that may follow. Standard therapy includes lifestyle modifications such as dietary compliance and weight loss, avoidance of trauma that leads to follicular rupture and active multimodal anti-inflammatory therapy. Given the importance of weight loss in the aims to resolve HS, bariatric intervention (both restrictive and malabsorptive) may be viewed as a means to achieve the drastic reduction in weight needed in patients who struggle to accomplish this without surgical intervention.

RISKS TO THE SKIN

While the aforementioned are examples of the positive effects of gastric bypass surgery on the skin, achieving radical weight reduction via an invasive bariatric procedure is not without inherent risks and complications. Bariatric surgery includes restrictive procedures such as laparoscopic banding, sleeves, and malabsorptive procedures including Roux-en-Y-gastric bypass (RYGB) and biliopancreatic diversion. The most common method is RYGB where an isolated portion of the stomach is directly connected to the small intestine, resulting in decreased gastric capacity, decreased acid secretion and diminished nutrient absorption. Bariatric surgery can be accompanied by micronutrient insufficiencies and metabolic imbalances that affect the skin. Such deficiencies can lead to changes in the skin's micro-architecture, which can, in turn, affect processes including wound healing. Changes in the skin's immune defense mechanisms can also result from vitamin and nutrient deficiency, increasing susceptibility to pathogens (Zouridaki 2014). The nutrient insufficiencies are presumed to be a result of a combination of decreased food intake, changes in the digestive system's anatomy, and high levels of oxidative stress that interfere with the absorptive process (Halawi 2013). The specific nutrition-related complications that will be detailed in this chapter include vitamin A, vitamin B3, biotin, vitamin C, iron, copper, vitamin K, and zinc. In attempt to prevent the dermatologic complications, post-bariatric patients are routinely prescribed dietary supplements to compensate for future insufficiencies. Interestingly, while patients may be compliant with their oral nutritional supplements, low circulating levels can still persist since the absorption is decreased. Recognizing various skin changes secondary to nutrient deficiency in post bariatric surgery patients is a valuable asset in providing comprehensive care.

Vitamin A

Vitamin A or retinol is a liposoluble vitamin found in foods derived from sources including cow's milk, liver, eggs, fish oils, mangos, tomatoes, and beta-carotene containing vegetables. Vitamin A is vital for optimum immune system function (Zalesin 2011; Jen 2010). Deficiency in retinol may be due to inadequate intake in patients with restricted diets or various metabolic alterations observed after gastric bypass procedures. These alterations include fat malabsorption, diminished protein absorption, and higher levels of oxidative stress. Interestingly, in developing countries, vitamin A-deficient children who were treated with augmented dietary protein intake demonstrated an increase in serum retinol levels (Zalesin 2011). This supports the intimate interaction between serum retinol and the carrier proteins that determine the bioavailability of serum retinol concentration. As such, total body stores of vitamin A may not truly be deficient but, rather, low levels of nutritional protein binding transport capacity may underlie these serum retinol findings.

Cutaneous findings classically observed include follicular and keratotic papules that usually affect the anterolateral surface of thighs and arms. This condition is known as phrynoderma and may also be associated with other vitamin deficiencies. The lesions may overtake the extensor surface of upper and lower limbs, shoulder, abdomen, dorsal area, buttocks and neck. Other dermatologic signs of vitamin A deficiency include: xeroderma, brittle or corkscrew hair, and thinning of the skin (Jen 2010). A correlation between low plasma vitamin A and E and the subsequent development of acne has also been speculated (El-Akawi 2006).

Diagnosis is made based on serum retinol levels, clinical evaluation, and positive response to treatment. Normal serum retinol levels range from 28 to 86 µg/dL (1 to 3 µmol/L). Levels, however, decrease only after the deficiency is advanced because the liver contains large stores of vitamin A. Therefore, when a deficiency is clinically suspected, a therapeutic trial of vitamin A may help establish the definitive diagnosis. Supplementation alone or in combination with other fat-soluble vitamins (D, E, and K) may be indicated in this setting. Current treatment recommendations are as follows: vitamin A palmitate in oil 60,000 international units (IU) orally once per day for two days, followed by 4500 IU orally once per day.

In summary, vitamin A deficiency remains an underreported postoperative complication of bariatric surgery. It is of paramount importance in the ongoing medical management of these patients that clinicians are aware of the cutaneous signs of retinol insufficiency. Furthermore, vitamin A deficiency should be suspected in those with protein-calorie malnutrition.

Vitamin B3

Vitamin B3 is converted to nicotinamide, a cofactor essential for cellular metabolism. In the intestine, the gut flora converts nicotinamide into nicotinic acid that is subsequently transported to the liver, kidneys and intestines. Sources of B3 include meat, poultry, nuts, eggs, fish, coffee and beans. Vitamin B3 is also synthesized in humans from the essential amino acid tryptophan. Pellagra, the classic triad of dementia, dermatitis and diarrhea, is the typical manifestation of vitamin B3 insufficiency. The dermatologic signs resemble a sun-burn on the affected areas. A symmetrical eruption of scaling and skin thickening, with a clear margin between the unaffected and affected skin, is classically observed. The dorsal aspect of the hands is the most affected site and may present in a glove-like distribution. Additionally, the skin lesions may also be noted around the neck; this is denoted as Casal's necklace (Jen 2010) (Figure 1). Other skin manifestations linked to niacin deficiency include glossitis and angular cheilitis, sulfur flakes over the nose, and a copper hue to affected skin (Burke 2013). The patient may report that the rash burns or is intensely itchy. Histopathological changes in the acute phase include subepidermal vesicle formation as a result of spongiosis, ballooning degeneration, and vacuolar alteration of the basal layer (Hegyi 2004).

It is critical for clinicians to remain vigilant in assessing for vitamin B3 deficiency in patients that have undergone gastric bypass. The diagnosis can be made by measuring urinary N-methyl-nicotinamide concentration. Alternatively, low 5-hydroxyindoleacetic acid (5-HIAA), a metabolite of serotonin, may also be an indication of niacin insufficiency. Pellagra can be devastating to the patient but is, fortunately, easily reversed with replacement therapy. Complications such as delirium, depression, dilated cardiomyopathy, and, ultimately, death can be prevented by prompt recognition and implementation of vitamin B3 replacement. Dietary niacin, however, may not be sufficient to maintain the body's needs over an extended period of time (Leklem 1991). The recommended daily allowance is around 16mg per day for adult males and 14mg per day for females. Treatment is usually oral nicotinoamide (100-200mg three times daily) until signs and symptoms resolve after several weeks of therapy (Crook 2014).

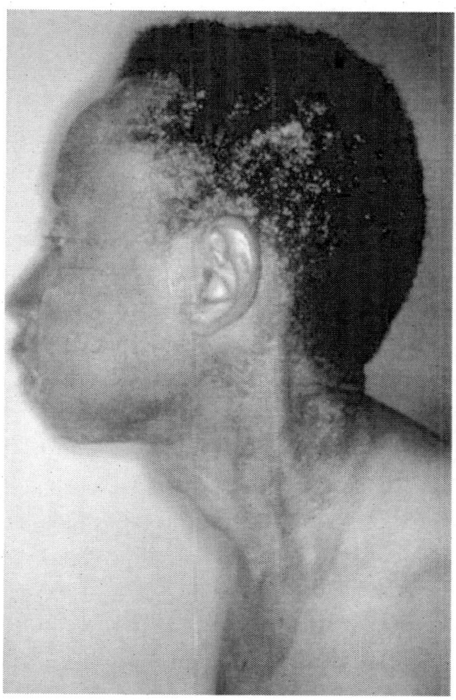

Figure 1. Casal's necklace of pellagra. Courtesy of Ron Grimwood, MD.

Biotin

Biotin, a cofactor for carboxylase synthetase enzymes, is absorbed in the small intestine. It is essential in the metabolism of carbohydrates, fats, and select amino acids. Furthermore, it is critical for proper cellular function, growth, and development. Additional studies have also suggested that biotin may play a role in glucose metabolism at the level of gene expression (Rodriguez 2003). Likewise, biotin is crucial in immune function and cell proliferation. Humans cannot synthesize biotin and, therefore, must obtain this vitamin from exogenous sources (i.e., nutrition and intestinal bacterial synthesis). Dietary sources of biotin include egg yolks, liver, nuts, peanuts, mushrooms, cow's milk, and soy (Mock 2000; Lanska 2012). Deficiency occurs in patients with a short gut or malabsorption. The classic cutaneous finding associated with biotin deficiency is an erythematous, scaling, crusting dermatitis present around the eyes, nose, mouth, and perineal region. The tongue may also be red and sore, and the hair is commonly fine and thinned (Balint 1998). Diagnosis is made on clinical grounds based on the presenting dermatologic findings, as well as response to replacement therapy. If left untreated, acquired biotin deficiency may ultimately result in hyperaesthesia, paraesthesia, depression, and muscle pain. It is important for physicians to be astute in initiating a trial of biotin if clinical suspicion of insufficiency is high and the patient has a known risk factor such as a history of gastric bypass. A dose of 10-40mg per day orally, or intramuscularly, is the current recommendation for therapeutic replacement.

Vitamin C

In addition to serving as a cofactor in the synthesis of carnitine and catecholamines (dopamine and norepinephrine), ascorbic acid has anti-oxidant properties, stabilizes vitamin E and folic acid, and, also, acts as a cofactor for the enzyme that catalyzes the formation of hydroxylysine and hydroxyproline. Flaws in the synthesis of hydroxylysine and hydroxyproline secondary to vitamin C insufficiency interfere with collagen synthesis, thus, impairing wound healing. Additionally, ascorbic acid is part of the metabolism of prostaglandins and prostacyclins which, when inadequately produced, can generate decreased inflammatory response and increased immunological susceptibility (Jen 2010).

Dietary sources include citrus fruits, strawberries, tomatoes, vegetables and potatoes. Absorption occurs in the upper third of the intestine. Scurvy is the most classic consequence of vitamin C deficiency. This insufficiency, therefore, is often diagnosed by dermatologists. The clinical manifestations tend to occur one to three months after the start of a vitamin-deficient diet. The first signs are fatigue, malaise, and lethargy. The "four Hs" are characteristic of scurvy: hemorrhagic signs, hyperkeratosis of hair follicles (on the lateral and posterior areas of the arms buttocks, and thighs), hypochondriasis, and hematologic abnormalities. Perifollicular petechiae are also a characteristic finding (Fossitt 2009). The main changes in the oral cavity are the presence of edematous, erythematous, and friable gingiva with tendency to bleeding (Li

2008). Hansen et al. report a case of a woman following gastric bypass who presented with painful swelling, bruising, and small ulcers on her lower extremities (Hansen 2012). Within 24 hours, she developed confluent purpuric plaques on the lower extremities and a sepsis-like condition. The diagnosis of vitamin C deficiency was based on the clinical picture in conjunction with a positive response to supplementation. The daily recommended supplementation is ascorbic acid, 800-1000mg per day given orally for a few days to one week and maintenance of 100mg per day. In cases where the diagnosis is uncertain, serum ascorbic acid levels may be confirmatory.

In summary, following bariatric surgery, patients are at risk of developing vitamin C deficiency, especially if the operation is combined with a poor diet. When spontaneous ecchymosis or petechiae are observed in at-risk patients, scurvy must be included in the differential. While untreated scurvy may be fatal, the symptoms of scurvy rapidly improve when the patient is treated with adequate doses of vitamin C.

Iron

Iron is a mineral found in all cells of the human body. Dietary sources include dried beans, fruits, egg yolks, liver, beef, oysters, salmon, whole grains, broccoli, spinach, and kale. The majority of iron absorption is carried out in the duodenal epithelium. Acidity and the presence of solubilizing agents like sugars facilitate the intestinal absorption. Reduced gastric acid secretion after a gastric bypass, therefore, can impair the absorption of iron in the duodenum. Additionally, after Laparoscopic Roux-en-Y Gastric Bypass (LRYGB) the duodenum is excluded from digestive continuity, further impairing iron absorption (Ruz 2009).

Iron is essential for a multitude of functions including oxygen transport, DNA synthesis, energy metabolism, and metabolism of collagen (Richardson 1996; Polefka 2012). Iron plays a critical role in the structure and function of skin. It aids in wound healing and protection against cellular damage secondary to reactive oxygen species. Exposure of skin fibroblasts to UVA can generate reactive oxygen species that promote oxidative damage in lysosomal, mitochondrial, nuclear, and plasma membranes. Ultimately, necrotic cell death will result due to the loss of plasma membrane integrity (Aroun 2012). As a transition metal which exists in two stable states, Fe^{2+} (electron donor) and Fe3+ (electron acceptor), iron plays a key role in preventing oxidative stress processes (Pelle 2011). Dermatologic manifestations of these effects are pallor, glossitis, koilonychia, angular cheilitis, and brittle hair and nails. Additionally, the tongue may become swollen and smooth and develop a burning sensation. Iron deficiency may also predispose one to bacterial and fungal infections, such as impetigo, boils and candidiasis (Jen 2010).

Obinwanne et al. performed a 10-year analysis of iron deficiency after laparoscopic Roux-en-Y Gastric Bypass (LRYGB) and reported an incidence of 53.1% (492 of 959 patients) (Obinwanne 2013). Furthermore, iron deficiency was more common in women, particularly those who were premenopausal or who had a history of abnormal uterine bleeding. According to the American College of Surgeons, female patients should be counseled that there is a 50% chance they will become iron deficient after LRYGB. Serum ferritin levels are assayed at three and six months postoperatively and then annually after the second postoperative year for those with initially low ferritin levels. Oral replacement is indicated if the patient has a postoperative ferritin less than 50 ng/mL and is administered in the following forms: ferrous gluconate, ferrous sulfate, ferrous fumarate, and ferrous bisglycinate. Oral iron therapy is limited after surgery due to decreased intestinal absorption (Mizon 2007). Another limitation of oral iron is that it is associated with significant gastrointestinal side effects that may ultimately lead to poor compliance. Common side effects include nausea, abdominal pain, diarrhea, and constipation. After a 3-month period of oral iron therapy, the ferritin level is assayed again. If it remains less than 50 ng/mL, the patient should be referred to the hematology clinic.

Indications for initiating intravenous (IV) iron therapy are poor tolerance of oral iron and poor response to oral iron treatment. IV iron treatment was required in 64 (6.7%) of the patients in the Obinwanne et al. study. The most commonly used form of IV iron was iron dextran (81.3%). This is largely because, unlike other forms, it is typically given as a single dose and does not require frequent visits to the hematology clinic. It is, therefore, the most cost-effective form of IV iron therapy. However, due to its association with rare, but serious, anaphylaxis, a test dose with premedication is recommended before infusion begins (Quinibi 2010; Defilipp 2013).

Iron deficiency is a problem that continues to cause complications in patients who have had gastric bypass. The aforementioned longitudinal study highlights the importance of strict postoperative follow-up of patients, with particular attention to those who may be at a higher risk for developing iron deficiency. Early detection of iron deficiency is key to the successful management of patients after gastric bypass.

Copper

Copper, a metal found in plasma, erythrocytes, cerebrospinal fluid, saliva, and gastric secretions, is obtained from the ingestion of meat, seafood, vegetables, grains, and nuts. Copper is an essential cofactor in many enzymatic reactions vital to the normal function of hematologic and vascular systems. Additionally, copper has a crucial role in direct and indirect antibacterial mechanisms as well as early wound healing (Griffith 2009; Mirastschijski 2013). Many patients with an acquired copper deficiency have a history of gastric surgery, even in the distant past (Prodan 2009). The proposed mechanism of copper deficiency is likely due to the decreased absorption in the stomach and proximal duodenum. Consequences of copper deficiency may manifest clinically dermatologically as poor wound healing, depigmented and thinning hair, and alopecia (Palint 1998). Copper deficiency does not manifest as dramatically on the skin as other micronutrient deficiencies, but a high level of suspicion should remain because it may accompany other deficiencies. Approximately 70% of women may experience some level of copper deficiency after gastric bypass. Early detection and treatment can prevent the hematologic and neurologic symptoms such as pancytopenia and myeloneuropathy, respectively.

Diagnosis is based on low levels of cerulopasmin and copper. These laboratory values, however, are not always accurate. Therefore, a positive response to supplementation may be the key in diagnosing the insufficiency. Treatment is usually in the form of copper sulfate 1.5-3mg per day given orally, but severe deficiencies may need to be replaced intravenously (Griffith, 2009).

Vitamin K

Dietary deficiency of vitamin K, a fat-soluble vitamin, is rare in adults because 50% of daily needs are synthesized by bacteria. Low vitamin K, however, may be seen in patients after undergoing malabsorptive procedures. Vitamin K is essential for the synthesis of several coagulation factors such as II, VII, IX, X, protein C, and protein S. Dietary vitamin K (phylloquinone) is found in green leafy vegetables, liver, brussel sprouts, lentils, plant oils, and soybeans. It is absorbed through active transport in the upper small intestine. The classic cutaneous findings secondary to vitamin K deficiency are related to the extravasation of blood into the skin manifested as purpura, petechiae, ecchymoses, and bruising (Jen 2010; Palint 1998). Clinically, it is important for physicians to be vigilant in investigating evidence of bleeding and bruising on the skin so as to prevent more severe and devastating hemorrhages.

Diagnosis is suspected based on routine coagulation study findings (prolonged prothrombin time or elevated international normalized ratio) and confirmed by a positive response to vitamin K administration. Some institutions may detect vitamin K deficiency more directly by measuring serum vitamin K levels (normal: 0.2-1.0 ng/ml). Vitamin K deficiency is typically treated orally, but, in the instance of fat malabsorption seen after bariatric interventions, intramuscular phytonadione 5-10 mg per day may be required.

Zinc

Bariatric surgery is a risk factor for developing a zinc deficiency. Zinc absorption occurs in the duodenum and proximal jejunum. It is these portions of the intestine that are bypassed in the RYGB procedure. Zinc is a primordial element essential to the structural and regulatory functions of over 200 enzymes. It can be found in most meat, legumes, whole grains, and dairy products. Its key role is in metabolic pathways, mediating immune function, cell replication, and DNA synthesis. Overall, zinc allows for the proper function of T-cells, neutrophils, natural killer cells, and proper wound healing (Kumar 2012; Vick 2015).

Due to this mineral's extensive roles in a multitude of biological processes, many systemic and dermatologic complications may manifest in the setting of moderate to severe deficiency. The classic clinical triad is comprised of diarrhea, alopecia, and acral and periorifacial rashes. This rash tends to be symmetrical, erosive, and eczematous. Other cutaneous features include vitiligo-like lesions, delayed wound healing, paronychia, stomatitis, psoriasiform dermatitis, angular cheilitis, and blepharitis (Kumar 2012).

Diagnosis is generally made by serum zinc levels below 50-70 µg/dL paired with recognition of the classic cutaneous findings (Krebs 2013). In cases of protein malnutrition experienced after surgery, there are changes in the intestinal structure and function with decrease in villi surface area culminating in a reduced capacity of zinc absorption. Moreover, it is likely that the decline in gastric secretion and the oxidative stress resulting from surgery also contribute to this diminished absorption of zinc. Ruz et al. studied the effects of zinc absorption in 56 morbidly obese women status post RYGB surgery. They measured mean plasma zinc, erythrocyte membrane alkaline phosphatase activity, and absorptive capacity of zinc. The percentage of absorption decreased significantly from 32.3% to 21% 18 months post-operation (Ruz 2011).

If left untreated, zinc deficiency has the potential to be lethal. Typical treatment of acquired zinc deficiency consists of elemental zinc 1-3mg/kg orally once daily until symptoms and signs resolve. Serum or plasma levels of zinc should be monitored during administration of oral replacement. Cutaneous findings will clinically improve prior to a significant change in serum levels. Additionally, copper levels should be monitored as high levels of zinc may lead to a reciprocal decrease in serum copper. Interestingly, Vick et al. reported a case of a woman who presented with a painful, pruritic vulvar rash despite 35mg of oral zinc replacement (Figure 2). The patient eventually had complete resolution of symptoms after two infusions of 2mg/kg per day of IV zinc. This highlights the fact that patients receiving malabsorptive procedures may not respond to traditional oral supplementation. Clinicians must be mindful of the fact that patients who have undergone structurally altering, malabsorptive surgeries may not respond to oral dietary supplementation, but rather require IV supplementation to resolve the consequences of the dietary insufficiency.

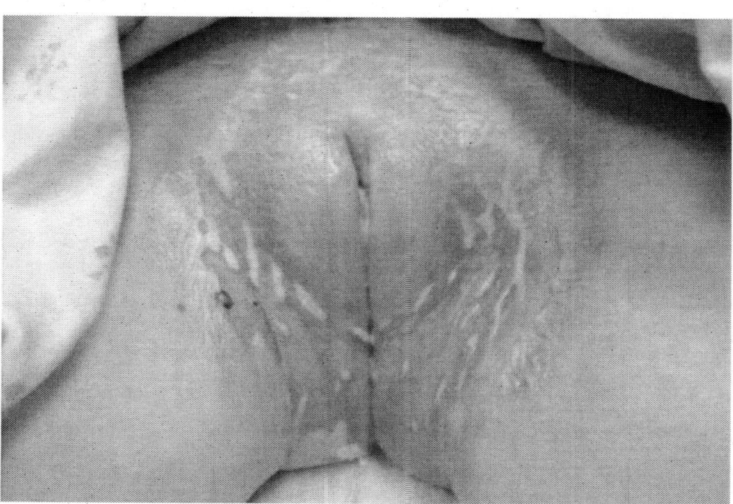

Figure 2. Perineal dermatitis of zinc deficiency. *Reprinted with permission* (Vick G, Mahmoudizad R, Fiala K. Intravenous therapy for acquired zinc deficiency secondary to gastric bypass surgery: a case report. Dermatologic Therapy; 2015. Wiley publisher).

CONCLUSION

In summary, bariatric surgery has significant value in aiding patients who are unable to lose weight without surgical intervention to achieve drastic weight loss. Additionally, the literature provides ample evidence that this weight loss, combined with alteration of hormones and inflammatory mediators, results in reduced comorbidities of obesity including chronic, refractory dermatologic conditions such as psoriasis, necrobiosis lipoidica, acanthosis nigricans, and hidradenitis suppurativa. Along with the various benefits, risks and the potential for serious complications are inherent as well. Patients who have a recent or remote history of gastric bypass surgery are prone to a myriad of dermatological manifestations related to skin inflammation or impaired ability to promote proper wound healing. Even after vitamin and nutrient replacement therapy, however, clinical improvement may not be completely sustained. This highlights the dynamic nature of nutrient insufficiencies and the clinical manifestations that follow. Given the current obesity epidemic and steadily rising number of bariatric procedures performed each year, knowledge of these dermatologic complications secondary to micronutrient deficiency is essential to the clinician's ability to provide comprehensive care, and, subsequently, improve the patient's quality of life.

REFERENCES

Aroun, A., Zhong, J. L., Tyrrel, R. M. et al. Iron, Oxidative stress and the example of solar ultraviolet a radiation. *Photochemical and Photobiological Sciences,* 2012 11, 118-134.

Atwa, M., Emara, A., Balata, M., et al. Serum leptin adiponectin and resistin among adult patients with acanthosis nigricans: correlations with insulin resistance and risk factors for cardiovascular disease. *International Journal of Dermatology,* 2014 53, 410-420.

Balint, J. Physical findings in nutritional deficiencies. *Pediatric clinics of North America,* 1998 45, 245-260.

Barbieri, R., Ryan, K. Hyperandrogenism, insulin resistance, and acanthosis nigricans syndrome: a common endocrinopahy with distinct pathophysiologic features. *American Journal of Obstetrics and Gynecology,* 1983 147, 90-101.

Bozkurt, S., Coskun, H., Kadioglu, H. et al. Remission of Ulcerated Necrobiosis Lipoidica Diabeticorum after Bariatric Surgery. *Case Reports in Dermatologic Medicine*, 2013, 352579-352579.

Burke, K., Adams, E. Nutritional Deficiency. *Directions in residency*, 2013, 1-2.

Crook M. The importance of recognizing pellagra (niacin deficiency) as it still occurs. *Nutrition, 2014* 30, 729-730.

Cruz, P., Hud, J. Excess insulin binding to insulin-like growth factor receptors: proposed mechanism for acanthosis nigricans. *Journal of Investigative Dermatology*, 1992 98, 82-85.

Defilipp, Z., Lister, J., Gagne, D. et al. Intravenous iron replacement for persistent iron deficiency anemia after Roux-en-Ygastric bypass. *Surgery for Obesity and Related Diseases*, 2013 9, 129-132.

El-Akawi, Z., Abdel-Latif, N., Abdul-Razzak, K. Does the plasma level of vitamins A and E affect acne condition. *Clinical and Experimental Dermatology*, 2006 31, 430-434.

Farias, M. M., Achurra, P., Boza, C. et al. Psoriasis following bariatric surgery: clinical evolution and impact on quality of life on 10 patients. *Obesity Surgery*, 2012 22, 877-80.

Faurschou, A., Zachariae, C. Gastric Bypass Surgery: Improving psoriasis through a GLP-1 dependent mechanism. *Medical hypotheses*, 2011 77, 098-1101.

Fossitt, D., Kowalski T. *Classic skin findings of scurvy.* Mayo Clinic Proceedings, 2014 89, 61.

Griffith, D. P., Liff, D. A., Ziegler, T. R. et al. Acquired copper deficiency: a potentially serious and preventable complication following gastric bypass surgery. *Obesity* (Silver Spring), 2009 17, 827-831.

Halawi, A., Abiad, F., Abbas, O. Bariatric surgery and its effects on the skin and skin diseases. *Obesity Surgery,* 2013 23, 408-413.

Hansen, E. P., Metzxche, C., Henningsen, E. et al. Severe scurvy after gastric bypass surgery and a poor postoperative diet. *Journal of Clinical Medical Research,* 2012 4, 135-137.

Hector, R. T., Aminian, A., Corcelles, R. Psoriasis Improvement After Bariatric Surgery. *Surgery for obesity and related diseases,* 2014 10, 1155-1160.

Hegyi, J., Schwartz, R., Hegyi, V. Pellagra: dermatitis, dementia, and diarrhea. *International Journal of Dermatology*, 2004 43, 1-5.

Holst, J. J. The Physiology of Glucagon-like Peptide 1. *Physiological Reviews*, 2007 87, 1409-1439.

Hossler, E. W., Wood, G. C., Still, C. D. et al. The effect of weight loss surgery on the severity of psoriasis. *British Journal of Dermatology,* 2013 168, 660-661.

Jen, M., Yan, A. Syndromes associated with nutritional deficiency and excess. *Clinics in dermatology,* 2010 28, 669-685.

Krebs, N. F. Update on zinc deficiency and excess in clinical pediatric practice. *Annals of Nutrition and Metabolism,* 2013 62, 19-29.

Kumar, P., Lal, N. R., Mondal, A. K. et al. Zinc and skin: a brief summary. *Dermatology Online Journal [eScholarship],* 2012 8.

Lanska, D. The discovery of niacin, biotin, and pantothenic acid. *Annals of Nutrition and Metabalism,* 2012 61, 246-253.

Leklem, J., Machlin, L. Handbook of Vitamins. 2nd ed. New York: Marcel Dekker., 1991.

Li, R., Byers, K., Walvekar, R. R. Gingival hypertrophy: a solitary manifestation of scurvy. *American Journal of Otolaryngology,* 2008 29, 426.

Margesson, L., Danby, F. Hidradenitis suppurativa. *Best Practice and Research Clinical obstetrics and Gynocology,* 2014 28, 1013-1027.

Mirastschijski, U., Martin, A., Jorgensen, L. N. et al. Zinc, copper, and selenium tissue levels and their relation to subcutaneous abscess, minor surgery, and wound healing in humans. *Biological Trace Element Research,* 2013 153, 76-83.

Mizon, C., Ruz, M., Csendes, A. et al. Persistent anemia after Roux-en-Y gastric bypass. *Nutrition,* 2007 23, 277-280.

Mock, D., Shils, M. *Modern Nutrition in Health and Disease.* 9th ed. Philadelphia: Lippincott Williams and Wilkins., 2000 459-459.

Obinwanne, K. M., Fredrickson, K. A., Mathiason, M. A. et al. Incidence, Treatment, and Outcomes of Iron Deficiency after Laproscopic Roux-en-Y Gastric Bypass: A 10-Year Analysis. *Journal of American College of Surgeons,* 2013 218, 246-252.

Palint, J. P. Physical Finding in Nutritional Deficiency. *Pediatric Clinics of North America,* 1998, 245-260.

Pasparakis, M. Regulation of tissue homeostasis by NF-kB signaling: implications for inflammatory diseases. *Nature Reviews Immunology,* 2009 9, 778-788.

Patsatsi, A., Kyriakou, A., Sotiriadis, D. Necrobiosis lipoidica: early diagnosis and treatment with tacrolimus. *Case Reports in Dermatology,* 2011 *3,* 89-93.

Pelle, E., Jian, J., Eclercq, L. et al. Protection against ultraviolet A-induced oxidative damage in normal human epidermal keratinocytes under post-menapausal conditions by an ultraviolet A-activated caged-iron chelator: a pilot study. *Photodermatology, Photoimmunology and Photomedicine,* 2011 27, 231-235.

Polefka, T. G., Bianchini, R. J., Shapiro, S. Interaction of mineral salts with the skin: a literature survey. *International Journal of Cosmetic Science,* 2012 34, 416-423.

Prodan, C. I., Bottomley, S. S., Vincent, A. S. Copper deficiency after gastric surgery: a reason for caution. *American Journal of the Medical Sciences,* 2009 337, 256-258.

Pugeat, M., Ducluzeau, P. H., Mallion-Donadieu, M. Association of insulin resistance with hyperandrogenia in women. *Hormone Research in Paediatrics,* 2000 54, 322-6.

Qunibi, W. Y. The efficacy and safety of current intravenous iron preparations for the management of iron-deficiency anemia: a review. *Arzneimittel-forschung,* 2010 60, 399-412.

Revuz, J. E., Gregor, B. E. Diagnosing hidradenitis suppurativa. *Dermatologic Clinics, 2016 34, 1-5.*

Richardson, D. R., Dickson, L., Baker, E Intermediate steps in cellular iron uptake from transferrin II. A cytoplasmic pool of iron is released from cultured cells via temperature-dependent mechanical wounding. *In Vitro Cellular and Developmental Biology - Animal,* 1996 32, 486-495.

Rodriguez-Melendez, R., Zempleni, J. Regulation of gene expression by biotin. *Journal of Nutritional Biochemisty,* 2003 14, 680-90.

Ruz, M., Carrasco, F., Rojas, P. et al. Iron absorption and iron status are reduced after Roux-en-Y gastric bypass. *American Journal of Clinical Nutrition,* 2009 90, 527-532.

Ruz, M., Carrasco, F., Rojas, P. et at. Zinc_absorption and zinc status are reduced after Roux-en-Y gastric bypass: a randomized study using 2 supplements. *American Journal of Clinical Nutrition,* 2011 94, 1004-1011.

Sehgal, V., Bhattacharya., S., Verma, P. Juvenile, insulin-dependent diabetes mellitus, type 1-related dermatoses. *Journal of the European Academy of Dermatology and Venereology,* 2011 25, 625-636.

Stuart, C., Peters, E., Prince, M. et al. Insulin resistance with acanthosis nigricans: the roles of obesity and androgen excess. *Metabolism,* 1986 35, 197-205.

Thomas, C., Gordon, K., Mortimer, P. Rapid resolution of hidradenitis suppurativa after bariatric surgical intervention. *Clinical Experimental Dermatology,* 2014 39, 315-317.

Vick, G., Mahmoudizad, R., Fiala, K. Intravenous Zinc Therapy for Acquired Zinc Deficiency Secondary to Gastric Bypass Surgery: A Case Report. *Dermatologic Therapy, 2015* 28, 222-225.

Weismann, K., Burns, D. *Skin disorders in diabetes mellitus.* Rook's Textbook of Dermatology, 2004, 106-157.

Zalesin, K., Miller, W., Franklin, B. et al. Vitamin A Deficiency after Gastric Bypass Surgery: An Underreported Postoperative Complication. *Journal of Obesity,* 2011 2011, 760-764.

Zouridaki, E., Papafragkaki D. K., Papafragkaki H. et al. Dermatological Complications after Bariatric Surgery: Report of Two Cases and Review of the Literature. *Dermatology,* 2014 228, 5-9.

INDEX

post-bariatric surgery, vii, 50, 55, 56, 73,
   77, 82, 85, 88, 89
psychological interventions, 1

R

resistance, 4, 9, 19, 20, 24, 26, 38, 40, 42,
   46, 50, 53, 57, 58, 60, 63, 65, 67, 68, 72,
   74, 75, 77, 86, 95, 112, 115
resistin, 9, 20, 21, 26, 27, 28, 33, 35, 38, 40,
   42, 43, 46, 112
risk factors, 43, 66, 69
Roux-en-Y gastric bypass (RYGB), v, vii,
   1, 2, 3, 4, 5, 6, 7, 8, 11, 12, 13, 14, 16,
   17, 18, 19, 21, 22, 50, 51, 52, 54, 55, 56,
   58, 59, 65, 73, 85, 91, 102, 107, 108,
   110, 114

S

SCFA(s), 49, 60, 67
secretin, 14
somatostatin, 9, 14, 18, 23, 27
stress, 97, 102, 103, 107, 110
symptoms, 109

syndrome, 28, 33, 36, 38, 40, 41, 45, 47, 58,
   63, 68, 81, 84, 94, 95

T

tissue, 7, 19, 20, 29, 31, 33, 57, 61, 68, 98,
   100, 101
transport, 109
type 2 diabetes, v, 49, 71, 87, 90, 92, 93, 94,
   95
tyrosine, 9, 10, 11, 13, 23, 24, 30, 36, 44,
   45, 47, 49, 53, 54, 55, 62

W

weight reduction, 43

β

β-cell dysfunction, 53, 72, 74, 77
β-cell function, 35, 50, 51, 52, 54, 56, 60,
   62, 72, 73, 74, 78, 79, 80, 81, 86